"God put an amazing healing pow[...]s book you will learn how to unlock the healing force within. Ginny has an amazing healing story, and she gets to the root cause factors involved in the development of cancer and other chronic diseases. She gives you a step-by-step process to address these issues and allow your body to heal! I highly recommend this book!"

Dr. David Jockers DNM, DC, MS
DrJockers.com and Author of The Keto Metabolic Breakthrough

"Ginny is a woman of strength, intelligence and great character, and I was proud to be one of her doctors in this journey. Her book is filled with practical advice for people with cancer and people who desire to lower their risk. It's filled with many hidden gems that make it an enjoyable and intriguing read."

Dr. Amber Passini, MD
Biogenesis Medical Center

"Ginny reveals the true nature and importance of the interaction between the spiritual, psychological, and material aspects of dealing with a health crisis. She reveals how we can walk with God through great difficulty, resulting in positive impact on mind, emotions, and will, and then bearing fruit in the body. As a pastor who counsels many people through crises like these, I heartily recommend her book."

Dr. Wallace Henley
Author and Senior Associate Pastor of Second Baptist Church, Houston, Texas

"I was blessed to be part of Ginny's care team. I affectionately referred to her as my Rock Star Patient because Ginny educated and empowered herself. She followed recommendations and turned her cancer journey into a heart project. The pearls in this book could benefit others greatly in their search for healing and vitality."

Dr. Kenna Brooke, ND
Founder, SoulSage.com

"With a transparent heart, personal experience and an engaging spirit, Ginny invites you on a journey—her journey and possibly yours as well. She takes readers by the hand and skillfully leads them toward the goal of preventing and beating cancer."

Dr. Tom Elliff
Author, pastor and former president, SBC International Mission Board

"Ginny helped lift my haze of confusion. With a biblical, integrative approach and well-documented research, her book provides a solid game plan for battling cancer and preventing recurrence."

Jann Barclift
Cancer survivor

"In 2010, my oncologist at MD Anderson and these eight steps turned around my stage 4 diagnosis. My oncologist believed my lifestyle changes complemented her efforts. This book has inspired me to fine tune my habits so I can make it another ten years and beyond with 'no evidence of disease'!"

Anne Buck
Stage IV aggressive breast cancer survivor

"As a breast cancer survivor, Ginny's book has definitely inspired me to turn my life upside down. She has walked the walk and exemplified her deep faith. I know this book will be light of hope to many as it was to me."

Denise Jones
Two-time breast cancer survivor

"As a cancer survivor, Ginny's book challenged, convicted and encouraged me. It gave me the well-researched plan I've been looking for to prevent recurrence. Anyone could benefit from the hope found within its pages."

Sherree Martin
Former missionary, occupational therapist and breast cancer survivor

"This book is such a useful tool for me, both personally and professionally. As a cancer survivor who is still battling and a trained nurse who is seeing more and more the great limitations of using only traditional pharmaceutical-based practice, I have learned so much from Ginny's journey. The wealth of resources she cites has greatly helped me to continue my fight more effectively and help others do the same."

Stacey Smith, RN, BSN

"Ginny is passionate about helping us live longer and healthier by making healthy, lifestyle choices. Stewardship of our bodies is a God-given gift. You can start making these changes today to enhance your quality of life, prevent cancer, or improve your chances of beating cancer. Her recommendations are evidence-based, practical and doable. Thank you my friend!"

Paula Hemphill
Two-time breast cancer survivor and wife of Dr. Ken Hemphill

"A perfect balance of faith, medicine, and common sense. Ginny has planted a beacon of hope—leading to God—that each of us can follow when dark times descend. More than that, she's equipped us with the ability to prevent those dark times by taking steps now to live a healthy lifestyle. Not only is this a book I will treasure, but I'll purchase it by the case to have on hand to bless others."

Edie Melson
Author and Director of Blue Ridge Mountains Christian Writers Conference

"Ginny's book is the life-giving gift of hope. She is a trustworthy guide providing a clear, concise, and do-able roadmap to health and wholeness. No matter the diagnosis, be assured you have a future and a hope."

PeggySue Wells
Bestselling author and concerned mom of seven

UNLEASH
YOUR GOD-GIVEN
HEALING
Eight Steps to Prevent and Survive Cancer

GINNY DENT BRANT

WESTBOW
PRESS®
A DIVISION OF THOMAS NELSON
& ZONDERVAN

This book is a work of non-fiction. Unless otherwise noted, the author and the publisher make no explicit guarantees as to the accuracy of the information contained in this book and in some cases, names of people and places have been altered to protect their privacy.

WestBow Press books may be ordered through booksellers or by contacting:

WestBow Press
A Division of Thomas Nelson & Zondervan
1663 Liberty Drive
Bloomington, IN 47403
www.westbowpress.com
844-714-3454

Because of the dynamic nature of the Internet, any web addresses or links contained in this book may have changed since publication and may no longer be valid. The views expressed in this work are solely those of the author and do not necessarily reflect the views of the publisher, and the publisher hereby disclaims any responsibility for them.

Any people depicted in stock imagery provided by Getty Images are models, and such images are being used for illustrative purposes only.
Certain stock imagery © Getty Images.

Unless otherwise noted, Scripture taken from the New King James Version®. Copyright © 1982 by Thomas Nelson. Used by permission. All rights reserved.

Scripture quotations marked (ESV) are from the ESV® Bible (The Holy Bible, English Standard Version®), copyright © 2001 by Crossway, a publishing ministry of Good News Publishers. Used by permission. All rights reserved.

Scripture quotations marked (NIV) are taken from the Holy Bible, New International Version®, NIV®. Copyright © 1973, 1978, 1984, 2011 by Biblica, Inc.™ Used by permission of Zondervan. All rights reserved worldwide. www.zondervan.com The "NIV" and "New International Version" are trademarks registered in the United States Patent and Trademark Office by Biblica, Inc.™

ISBN: 978-1-9736-8812-9 (sc)
ISBN: 978-1-9736-8811-2 (hc)
ISBN: 978-1-9736-8848-8 (e)

Library of Congress Control Number: 2020904730

Print information available on the last page.

WestBow Press rev. date: 03/16/2020

Written in gratitude to a loving God, who made our bodies to heal and has provided so many healing agents in nature.

To my husband, Alton, my Tin Man, who always had a heart and loved me unconditionally through the toughest journey of my life.

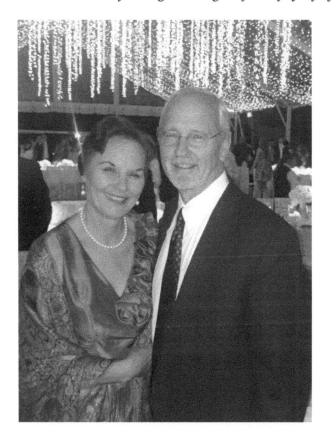

This book is for those who want to prevent cancer or recurrence, for those who must endure the journey, and for every caregiver who loves them.

And this is the book I never wanted to write!

CONTENTS

Foreword xiii

Acknowledgments xv

Introduction xvii

Chapter 1   Risk Factors: What about This Baptist Lifestyle? 1

Step One: Water
Chapter 2   Hydrating Your Body 13

Step Two: Sleep
Chapter 3   Restoring and Rebuilding Your Body with Deep Sleep ... 27

Step Three: Exercise
Chapter 4   Moving Your Body toward Optimum Health 39

Step Four: Nutrition
Chapter 5   Food as Powerful Medicine 57
Chapter 6   Fats, Gluten, Dairy, and Sugar 72
Chapter 7   Organics, Herbs, Oils, and Supplements 82

Step Five: Managing Stress
Chapter 8   Living Your Faith to Manage Stress and Emotions 99
Chapter 9   God's Remedies for Healing Emotions 113

Step Six: Thankfulness
Chapter 10   Practicing Gratitude as an Attitude 127

Step Seven: Detoxification

Chapter 11   Reducing Environmental Toxins 139

Chapter 12   Detoxing to Reduce Your Toxic Load 155

Chapter 13   The Invisible Toxin 167

Step Eight: Healing the Gut

Chapter 14   Restoring Your Microbiome 177

If You're on the Pink Brick Road...

Chapter 15   For Breast and Estrogen-Fed Cancer Only 191

Destination: Emerald City

Chapter 16   Promoting Longevity while Anticipating Heaven 211

Afterword 223

Notes 239

FOREWORD

I am honored to write the foreword for Ginny Brant's book about accepting the challenge of a cancer diagnosis and taking dedicated steps to beat it. A cancer diagnosis is devastating news for any person. It is for most people something that happens to "someone else." The moment a person receives the news immediately causes a cascade of immunosuppressive emotions such as fear, anxiety, stress, anger, and denial. The person's first thought is often, *Am I going to die? What about my family? My job? My dreams?*

This book is the result of one woman's cancer journey. Through courage, faith in God, and being proactive in battling the disease, Ginny survived this difficult journey. She did it by seeking out and taking the necessary steps to achieve victory. Now she has been called by God to share these steps with other cancer victims to help *them* navigate the ups and downs and twists and turns of this journey. These steps also help anyone who desires to prevent cancer.

In these pages you will read something of Ginny's personal cancer story, including the initial shock, the ensuing fear, the difficult medical decisions, her treatment plan, and how it all impacted her. But keep in mind that this was *her* journey, and your journey is only yours. Each cancer is different and unique to each individual. With breast cancer, even the same cell type may have a different tumor biology, stage, and genetic mutations. Your journey may be similar and yet be totally unique to you.

Your main goal is to achieve complete remission. Ginny has provided you with a tremendous roadmap involving eight powerful steps to help you reach that destination. I like all of these steps, but I ask that you give special attention to those involving hydration, rest, exercise, using food as medicine, relying on your faith to manage stress, and healing the gut.

As you read this book, be strengthened and encouraged. Don't get lost in the details of the science, but stay focused on what applies to you. Hear and receive the core message of each step without putting undue pressure on yourself to completely implement every suggestion. Do not feel guilty if you cannot follow each step totally, but commit yourself to be disciplined, keep a positive attitude, and engage in daily prayer. If you are diligent in implementing these eight steps to the best of your ability, they will help you to unleash the God-given healing within you.

God Bless,

Dr. Robert L. Elliott, MD, PhD, DSc
Director of the Elliott–Elliott–Head Breast Cancer Research
and Treatment Center in Baton Rouge, LA
Surgical oncologist, medical researcher, and owner of several cancer patents
Adjunct Clinical Associate Professor of Surgery, Medicine, and Biochemistry
at Tulane University Medical School

ACKNOWLEDGMENTS

A special thanks to my "wizard of an editor," David Webb, whose wisdom and experience has only enhanced this book. I also want to thank my tribe of friends who offered editing advice and encouraging support throughout the writing of this book: Stacey Smith, Chris Jarrard, April Warner, Pam Boller, Sharon Dillman, Tracie Dent, and Carol Montgomery.

I will always be grateful to the many doctors, naturopaths, nutritionists, nurses, technicians, and even drivers who poured their gifts into me and offered prayers and words of encouragement. Your caring service and willingness to serve me during my years of need are greatly appreciated. Special recognition goes to:

Dr. Kenna Barber, Naturopath
Dr. Miral Amin, Surgical Oncologist
Dr. Daniel Lui, Reconstructive Surgeon
Dr. Nimish Patel, Radiologist
Kimberly Randolph, Nurse Practitioner
Dr. Christopher Stephenson, Internist
Dr. John Schuler, Family Medicine
Dr. Ritwick Panicker, Oncologist
Dr. Amber Passini, MD
Colleen Mooney, Dietician

Finally, many thanks to all those who offered help and prayed for me through my journey.

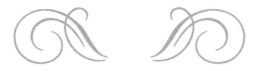

INTRODUCTION

The Unexpected Journey

Fight the good fight of faith, lay hold on
eternal life, to which you were also
called and have confessed the good confession
in the presence of many witnesses.
—1 Timothy 6:12

Ten months earlier, while visiting my eighty-two-year-old mother in Columbia, SC, she broke the shocking news to my husband and me: "I have breast cancer." With a twinkle in her eye she added, "This may be my ticket to heaven." Cancer had already spread throughout her body like a twister ravaging a Kansas farm.

"Oh my," I managed to say, selfishly not wanting to let her go. But I knew that twinkle meant, *I'm soon to enter the gates of heaven to bond with my Savior and see my soul mate, Harry, again.*

Over the next few months, I watched my mother endure the humiliation of the removal of her breasts. Through each trial, including medication that robbed her of her strength and femininity, she continued to whisper, "Heaven soon."

Following a double mastectomy and a daily regimen of hormone blockers, her cancer disappeared, and we sensed a reprieve. Several months later, however, cancer reappeared in her right hip bone. After several new rounds of radiation sent pain shooting throughout her abdomen, the radiologist prescribed IV fluids and pain medication.

Then I got a call from my sister, Dolly. "Her pain has increased," she said in desperation. "She needs to go to the emergency room." Hours later, Dolly called again. "It's serious. To save her life, they must remove the blockage and her large intestine. They're not sure she can survive the surgery."

When my mother heard the doctor's prognosis, she abruptly said, "No more surgeries."

I immediately drove to Columbia, realizing this might be it. When I arrived, my mother's belly was distended, probably from the radiation. She looked nine months pregnant. My family gathered around her bedside, looking to each other for answers. If things remained the same, she would soon realize her heart's desire and go to heaven.

As I stayed by her bedside one evening, she awakened and said, "Who's keeping me from going to heaven?" She fired a cold glance at the nurses, then her eyes locked on mine. "Ginny Dent Brant, you know my wishes. Whatever machine is keeping me alive, turn it off." I knew what she meant. Nothing was to keep her alive when there was no hope. Comfort only. Those were her wishes.

The next morning, her doctor came in. "I heard about your mother's request last night. I'm reversing her orders. We'll allow her to die a natural death and give comfort as needed."

The next forty-eight hours were the longest of my life as I watched every system in her body shut down one at a time. I'd been there before with my dad. My mom held on until the last of her grandchildren came to say goodbye. My son Jonnie was the last to arrive. As she sensed the tears flowing down his cheeks, she said, "It's okay. Death is a part of life. I've been blessed by all of you. See you in heaven."

Each of her children honored this great woman with a eulogy at her memorial service. During my eulogy, I sang one verse from the old spiritual "Swing Low, Sweet Chariot." My mother had transitioned to her eternal reward—that place over the rainbow.

A Bump in the Night

Five months later, still grieving the loss, my husband, Alton, and I celebrated our good health by taking part in the Cooper River Bridge Run in Charleston along with 45,000 other participants.

The next evening, I awakened in the middle of the night when my ring became entangled in my nightgown. As I struggled to free it, my left hand brushed against my right breast.

There was a noticeable bump.

I took a few seconds to examine it. Oh well, I thought, I've had cysts before that proved to be nothing. I drifted back into my dreams.

The next day I scheduled a visit with my doctor, whom I'd just seen four months earlier. During my appointment, she felt the lump right away. She immediately arranged for a mammogram and ultrasound.

"I'm pretty sure it's a fluid-filled cyst," I offered casually.

The next week, during testing, I helpfully informed the mammogram technician, "It's in the right breast at seven o'clock."

"Oh, yes," she said. "You can't miss it."

"It's a fluid-filled cyst," I told her. "I've had them before."

She quickly moved me to the next room where another technician would do the ultrasound. I knew we could clear up this confusion in a jiffy. As the technician smeared cold jelly across my right breast, I told him, "I'm the queen of getting fluid-filled cysts."

"We'll see," he said.

Ten minutes later, the radiologist appeared. "It's not fluid-filled," he said. "It's solid."

"Really!" I said, catching my breath. "What percentage of these things is malignant?"

"Only one out of three," he said.

"So two out of three chances, it's nothing," I said, looking for assurance.

"That's right. We'll need a biopsy to determine for sure what it is."

The ultrasound finding had stunned me, but I was encouraged that the odds were in my favor. As all my friends knew, I was a health nut. Every time I'd had a risk factor screening with my yearly mammogram, I scored in the lowest-risk category.

I went to an oncologist in Greenville to set up my biopsy. As I drove into the cancer center parking lot, I prayed, "Lord, don't let this be." I hesitantly walked into the foreboding place, passing by the shadows of women with scarves replacing what once were locks of hair, and I shivered. With each step, dark glimmers of my mother's own cancer journey flashed before me.

The oncologist asked about family history, and I told him about my mom's cancer. "Well," he said, "if it's cancer, we've caught it early. A lumpectomy and a little radiation, and you'll be good to go."

The biopsy took longer and was far more painful than I expected. I felt as though I had been hit with a stun gun. I remember the radiologist saying, "It's movable and that's a good sign." I held on to those words.

I drove to work with ice layered on my breast. Our district superintendent had been holding down the fort until my arrival because the principal and assistant principal were out that week. I assured him everything was okay.

After lunch, I retreated to the high-security room where two thousand student tests served as a cloud of witnesses to the waves of emotion emanating from my chest. It was my job to sort these tests while protecting the integrity of the testing process, and I needed to be in the moment.

Only one out of three are malignant, I kept reminding myself, and most are benign.

When I arrived home that night, my husband greeted me with open arms. "It's going to be okay," he said. "You're not the cancer type."

Denial Turns into Reality

After forty-eight hours of waiting, I was beginning to sweat. I clung desperately to the hope that if this was cancer, we'd caught it early. Either way, I wanted this lump removed from my body; it was beginning to exercise control over my thoughts and emotions.

The next day, I was in the secure testing room again when I received a call from the oncologist's nurse. "Your results are back," she said. "It's cancer. And it's invasive."

I stopped sorting tests. "No, it can't be," I murmured.

"Ductal," she continued. "It's in the ducts. We won't know until next week what kind of cancer it is."

My world came to a standstill. In the blink of an eye, all my plans and dreams for the future were dangling in midair. I struggled to move or think.

I left school early that day. I did not pass go. I did not collect $200. I went straight home. I called my husband on the way. "Honey, it's cancer," I said. "I'm not the two out of three. It's real."

"Whatever happens," Alton said, "we'll face this together. You'll be fine. It's got to be early." When I arrived home, my husband wrapped his arms around me and held me as though the wind might sweep me away. I found comfort in his arms.

"Oh, Father," he prayed, "guide us through this journey. Give us wisdom, and may we glorify You in all that we do. I bring my precious wife and her healing of this cancer before Your throne. In Jesus's name, amen."

A week later I was in the testing room when the nurse called again. "Your results are in," she said. "Your cancer was driven by both estrogen and HER2." In some breast cancers, the cells make too much of a protein called HER2. "The HER2 means it's aggressive," she continued. "We'll need to set you up for a consult with a surgeon."

The news drove deep into my heart. I'd thought it was incomprehensible that I had cancer, and now I had to swallow the bitter pill that it was aggressive and life-threatening. The nurse assured me that every weapon would be brought to bear to save my life, but I knew those treatments were the medical equivalent of weapons of mass destruction.

Paula Hemphill, a friend and former International Mission Board trustee, was a survivor of HER2 breast cancer. She assured me that the cancer was survivable, but the road to recovery would be long. I began to google the drug Herceptin, which would be used to combat my cancer. For Paula, it was the miracle drug that saved her life. To me, it was a drug that could potentially damage my heart and lungs. Even if I survived, what would life be like after?

I felt trapped, with no way out. I desperately longed to return to the days before my diagnosis. My mind refused to grasp what was happening to my body. I wanted to wake up from this nightmare.

Paula assured me, "There *will* be life after cancer for you."

One day, while driving to Clemson with my husband, I said to him, "I feel as though God is giving me a gift, but it's a gift I don't want."

"I don't want it either." Alton chuckled. "But we'll face this together."

Second Opinions Matter

During my next visit with the surgeon, he noted that I had a large hematoma—a solid swelling of clotted blood—from the biopsy. The next step was to order an MRI, which would reveal the clearest picture and determine the extent of the surgery needed. My mind began to race with uncertainties. Could there be more tumors? Were my lymph nodes involved? Where would this nightmare end?

While driving to church one morning, Alton said, "I want a second opinion. This is serious stuff. I want to make sure we make the right decisions." We knew from my mom's experience that dealing with this cancer beast involved many tough decisions.

I remembered seeing the Cancer Treatment Centers of America (CTCA) booth at the National Religious Broadcaster's convention and gave them a call. Alton and I had an interesting conversation on speakerphone with one of their intake consultants. CTCA had centers in Atlanta, Chicago, Tulsa, Philadelphia, and Phoenix. Their second opinion would involve a surgeon, oncologist, radiologist, nutritionist, and naturopathic doctor. I didn't know then that CTCA supplemented chemotherapy, radiation, and surgery with integrative medicine. I was a big proponent of integrative medicine, which combines nutrition, nutraceuticals, and lifestyle changes along with conventional medicine to fight disease.

I called my former integrative medical doctor, Dr. Connie Ross, and asked her opinion on where to go for my second opinion. The first words out of her mouth were "CTCA in Chicago. If it were me, that's where I would go."

My husband and I prayed diligently that God would guide our steps, and we felt a peace about going to Chicago.

I went to work Monday morning with my suitcase in hand. CTCA had scheduled us to fly up that night for a series of appointments throughout the week. The last-minute arrangement of these appointments was a loving reminder that God knew my situation and was graciously paving our way. I didn't realize how significant a second opinion could be. If insurance pays for it, it's wise to get one, especially for a serious medical condition.

Before our flight, however, I met with the surgeon in Greenville to get the results of my MRI. That afternoon he gave me the worst news yet: The MRI showed an additional tumor, possible lymph node involvement, and activity in my upper torso.

That night we boarded a plane bound for Chicago. We were on our way to CTCA, or as my husband called it, Cancerville—the place where hurting, frightened people begin their journey in search of a cure. There's one sure truth about cancer: No one wants to get it. No one thinks they are going to get it. But whether we wanted it or not, Cancerville was our next destination.

The Magic Kingdom

Neither of us slept well that night. The news from my MRI boggled our minds. The next morning, our shuttle driver sang songs on our thirty-minute jaunt to Cancerville. As he rounded the corner to the entrance, he announced, "Here we are at the Magic Kingdom! Have a nice day and may God guide and bless your way."

Magic Kingdom, huh? I had been hoping for better news, an easier path. But this wasn't the Emerald City. This was Munchkinland, and I knew that I had a long, difficult journey ahead of me. But I also knew I was a child of the King of Kings. He had brought me to this place, and He was with me. To sense His presence in our deepest struggles, our toughest trials—it's magical and indescribable.

"Welcome to CTCA," said the doorman. "How may I help you?" He directed us to the registration desk. Everything ran like clockwork, and it was only a matter of minutes before we were meeting with our intake physician, Dr. Michael Delatorre.

"I didn't sleep well last night," I admitted.

"I understand," he replied. "I've looked at your background and medical tests. We've already read the slide from your biopsy. We concur that you do have breast cancer, which is driven by both estrogen and HER2. This afternoon you will have heart tests to clear you for the use of Herceptin."

Just the word *Herceptin* unnerved me. "Many people are calling it the Miracle Drug," I said. "But I read that Herceptin can damage your heart and lungs. I'm a very active person, and those two organs are dear to me. I'm not sure I can take that drug."

"Only 5 percent of patients experience heart or lung damage," he said compassionately. "First, we'll see if your heart is working properly. An echocardiogram will give us an Ejection Fraction (EF) rate. If your EKG is normal and your EF is 65 or above, you're cleared for Herceptin. It's standard procedure to recheck your EF every few months while you're on Herceptin."

"What about my MRI?" I asked. "My imaging appeared to be impersonating a tornado."

"I saw your MRI. Don't jump off the bridge yet," he said. "I've asked two surgeons and two radiologists to examine it and give me their opinions by tomorrow morning. If your tumor is that large, we can choose the option of doing the chemotherapy first. We have chemos that can melt that tumor or significantly shrink it before surgery."

"Really?"

"I also want to order some blood work. And you will meet with a surgeon, plastic surgeon, radiologist, oncologist, naturopathic doctor, and nutritionist. On Friday, we'll give you our plan. You'll be involved in deciding how we proceed."

Alton and I both appreciated this. We wanted to be involved.

The next day, we hurried to Dr. Delatorre's office, anxious to hear the opinion of the surgeons and radiologists. Alton gently held my hand as we waited. (I highly recommend handholding, whether in love or fear.)

"The doctors have reviewed your MRI," the doctor said. "They all agree that the enlarged tumor and tornado-appearing mass *may* not actually be cancer, but inflammation caused by a biopsy that went bad. It happens to some patients. Yours is one of the worst I've seen. You're fortunate your body was able to handle the massive inflammation."

Every cell in my body breathed a sigh of relief, then I asked, "You mean the cancer has not spread to my lymph nodes or upper torso?"

"We'll only know for sure after the lymph nodes are tested after surgery. Your tumor may have only enlarged due to inflammation. The inflammation in your upper body appeared as cancer on the MRI."

He continued. "They also noted they could see cancer on both previous years' mammograms. You have dense breasts, which makes reading a mammogram more difficult.

"After lunch, I've scheduled another biopsy to see if the new tumor is malignant. Dr. Patel will also examine your lymph nodes with an ultrasound to determine if the swelling is due to inflammation or cancer."

I shuddered at just the mention of another biopsy. "Will it hurt like before and swell that much? My entire breast was black and blue from the first one."

"No, it's not likely to happen again. Dr. Patel is very gentle. What happened to you is rare," he said.

There was a slight hope of reprieve. I had a skip in my walk as we left his office and headed to the cafeteria. I chose wild salmon with asparagus.

I looked at my husband and said, "What's the difference between wild salmon and the farm-raised salmon I've been eating?" Boy, did I have a lot to learn. The answer is chemicals.

Then I wondered aloud, "How did two previous mammograms miss my cancer? If caught earlier, I'd be in a better place!"

"Don't think about it, honey," my husband said. "God only gives us what we can handle. It may have been too much for you to handle during your mother's cancer."

After lunch, I underwent the biopsy. This one was so different from the first—little swelling and only a small bruise. What a difference! *Thank you, Lord!* I hugged Dr. Patel's neck.

Next, we met the surgical oncologist, Dr. Miral Amin. She was a ray of sunshine as she darted into my room in a knee-high skirt and boots. She measured my breasts with precision.

"I'm trying to determine if I can surgically remove the main tumor, and the secondary tumor if malignant, and still clear the margins," she said. "We'll know the results of your second biopsy in two days."

Breast conservation is the main goal of surgeons these days. This woman was determined to save my breast. She was honest with me and warned, "If I'm not able to clear the margins, a mastectomy will be needed."

CTCA provides a pathologist on site for surgeries such as mine to guide the surgeon as they remove tissue around the cancer. The final decisions are made when the tissue is processed with specific dyes and then viewed under a microscope.

I felt comfortable with Dr. Amin. Compassion and kindness seemed a natural part of her persona. She outlined three choices for me: extended lumpectomy (if possible) followed by radiation after chemo, mastectomy with no radiation, or double mastectomy. All three options included lymph node dissection.

My husband and I mulled over our options. "Lord, guide us to the right treatment and give us wisdom to make the right decisions," we prayed. Decisions, decisions, decisions.

After an organic breakfast of omelets, fresh fruit, and coffee, we met with oncologist Dr. Rakhshanda Neelam and her team. It was clear from her demeanor and insistence that chemotherapy would be a necessary part of my treatment. She gave me written information on the chemotherapies and their possible side effects.

The skip in my walk vanished.

Just glancing through the pages turned my digestive system upside down. The possible side effects included nausea, vomiting, fever, chills, leukemia, nerve damage, heart damage, brain damage, lung damage, kidney and liver failure, even death.

Wake up. Please wake up, I thought.

The best part of my visit that day was consulting with the nutritionist, Colleen Mooney. When she entered the room, I could no longer hold back the dam on my emotions. Colleen held my hand as I sobbed. "I'm here to make things better," she said.

"I don't understand why I got this cancer."

"Don't be too hard on yourself. Sometimes it just happens." Then she handed me a brochure and carefully explained the foods she wanted me to emphasize and the foods I would need to avoid during treatment.

"I never wanted chemo," I told her, wiping my tears.

"I know. We are going to do everything we can nutritionally to help you get through it."

She then introduced me to Dr. Khara Lucius, the naturopathic doctor on Dr. Neelam's team. Integrative and naturopathic medicine had helped me through a number of health issues in my life. I believed in using God's provisions found in nature and treating the root causes of disease.

Dr. Lucius assured me that she would also help me through the journey. "I'll provide nutrients and supplements to assist your healing after surgery, minimize the side effects of chemo, and protect you during radiation."

My tears subsided. God had given me two good fairies to guide and protect me on my journey down the Yellow Brick Road.

Finding Peace in Decisions

In a few days, I received the second biopsy results. "Ginny, it's Dr. Amin. The second tumor is also malignant, but I've measured down to the centimeter. I believe I can get both tumors and clear all the margins without doing a mastectomy. We have an opening for surgery in ten days. If you decide to allow us to do your surgery, you'll need to fly up the

Thursday before surgery for pre-op and meet with the plastic surgeon. How do you feel about that?"

"It's a good plan," I responded.

Although a bit of bad news, I trusted Dr. Amin. I trusted CTCA.

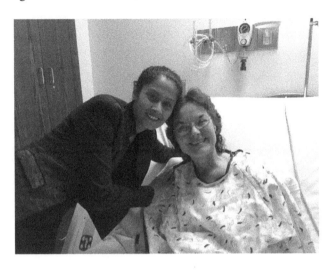

Dr. Miral Amin, my surgeon, holds a special place in my heart.

Most of all, I trusted God. I was so thankful to Him. *He* knew what I needed *before* my diagnosis. *He* was guiding my way, and *He* had never left my side.

There was no denying CTCA in Chicago was part of God's plan. I found it was not the Cancerville I had expected it to be. I was drawn to their integrative approach, personalized nutrition therapy, and vitamin C infusions. Their personalized care and customer service were magical—like Chick-fil-A on steroids. Alton and I both had a peace about it. Every cancer patient needs to feel a peace about the direction and treatments they take. Whatever they may be.

CTCA became my home away from home. Just being there gave me hope. I was ready to move forward.

A twister had swept through my life and set me on the path to Emerald City in search of a cure for my cancer. I wasn't in Kansas anymore. But I was ready to fight the good fight.

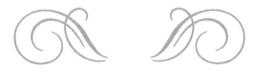

CHAPTER 1

Risk Factors: What about This Baptist Lifestyle?

Therefore we do not lose heart. Even though our outward man is perishing, yet the inward man is being renewed day by day. For our light affliction, which is but for a moment, is working for us a far more exceeding and eternal weight of glory, while we do not look at the things which are seen, but at the things which are not seen. For the things which are seen are temporary, but the things which are not seen are eternal.
—2 Corinthians 4:16–18

According to the American Cancer Society, one out of every two men will be diagnosed with some type of cancer in their lifetimes, and one of every three women. And the risk is only increasing. According to the World Health Organization, the number of new cases is expected to rise by about 70 percent over the next two decades.[1] Cancer has become as common as tornadoes in Kansas. It's time we wake up, face the reality, and develop a plan of prevention.

Family Risk Factors

I was thirty years old when my mother was diagnosed with colon cancer. My father had been diagnosed the year before with the same cancer. Thankfully, both cancers were discovered early and were remedied by surgery with no chemotherapy or radiation. Both cancers were discovered during routine colonoscopies, so my family believes in colonoscopies. I had my first such test that same year.

Imagine a doctor telling you at age thirty, "You're at high risk for colon cancer. If you don't have regularly scheduled colonoscopies, I can tell you what will be on your tombstone." That's when I first became proactive about preventing cancer. Honestly, I had already put myself at risk of developing skin cancer from decades of overexposure to the sun while sunbathing.

The Connection between Alzheimer's and Cancer

At age sixty-six, my father began showing signs of mental decline. At first, we just thought it was the result of normal aging, but when his personality began to change, we realized we were losing him to Alzheimer's disease. It was the beginning of a painful journey—one I would never want to experience again.

I began studying everything I could about Alzheimer's, and I learned that it may be caused by one's lifestyle as much as aging or genetics. When my mother and I were invited to attend the 2002 Alzheimer's and Cancer Medical Research Convention at the Omni in Charleston, SC, we eagerly attended. I'll never forget a slide one medical researcher presented. It clearly showed that as the chemicals and toxins in the environment increase and the immune system's strength decreases with age, there is a greater risk for diseases such as Alzheimer's and cancer.

What I learned at that convention changed my life. These doctors admitted they were not close to finding a cure for Alzheimer's. The only hope was prevention. Cancer research has developed many treatments, but prevention still offers the best hope for a cure. That doctor's prescription was clear—a healthy lifestyle of exercise, hydration, and lots of fruits and vegetables. "Fruits and vegetables contain antioxidants, which help to neutralize the free radicals that get into our bodies," he said.

Despite President Richard Nixon's War on Cancer in 1971, we've not stemmed its growth. Cancer rates have steadily increased. The medical profession continues to discover better ways to identify each type of cancer and provide more effective treatments and surgeries. But our inability to stop increasing cancer rates would seem to indicate that, although we've won some major battles, we are losing the war. In the 1930s, one in thirty Americans was diagnosed with cancer.[2] As chemicals in food, water, and the environment have increased, so have cancer diagnoses. Today's cancer rate is approaching one in two.[3]

I believe in the old adage "An ounce of prevention is worth a pound of cure." That's why I've always kept up with yearly mammograms and doctor visits. Obviously, I was not preventative enough.

The Risk Factors for Cancer

According to the American Cancer Society (ACS), the following are important lifestyle risk factors for cancer. The first five are risk factors that pertain to all cancers. The next five particularly relate to breast cancer.[4]

1. Drinking Alcohol

Excessive alcohol consumption is known to increase the risk of all cancers. Women who consume two to five drinks daily have about one and a half times the risk of getting breast cancer than women who don't drink alcohol. The ACS recommends that women have no more than one alcoholic drink a day. Men are limited to two. Some doctors recommend that their patients not partake of alcohol at all due to the risks.

2. Maintaining a Healthy Weight

The risk of all cancers increases with excess weight and obesity. Being overweight after menopause increases breast cancer risk. Before menopause, your ovaries produce most of your estrogen, while fat tissue produces a minimal amount. After menopause, most of a woman's estrogen comes from fat tissue. Excess fat tissue after menopause can raise estrogen levels and increase your chances of developing breast cancer. Also, women who are overweight tend to have higher blood insulin levels, which have been linked to several cancers.

It is recommended that you maintain a healthy weight throughout your life by balancing your food intake with physical activity. Estrogen and toxins are stored in adipose tissue (fat cells), so beware! Our body systems function much more efficiently when we maintain a healthy weight for our bone structure and height.

3. Physical Activity

Evidence is mounting that physical activity in the form of exercise reduces risk for all cancers. The ACS recommends that adults get at least 150 minutes of moderate intensity or seventy-five minutes of vigorous intensity activity every week.

4. Smoking

Smoking is a risk factor for every type of cancer—especially cancer of the lung, mouth, tongue, and esophagus. In recent years, more studies have shown that heavy smoking over a long period of time is linked to a higher risk of breast cancer.

5. Age

The risk factor for developing any type of cancer increases with age. Persons age sixty and older have the greatest susceptibility, with risk increasing every subsequent year.

6. Not Having Children

Women who have not given birth, or who had their first child after age thirty, are at a slightly higher risk for breast cancer. Having numerous pregnancies and becoming pregnant at an early age reduces breast cancer risk.

7. Birth Control

Studies have found that women using birth control pills have a slightly higher risk of breast cancer than women who have never used them. When considering the use of oral contraceptives, women should discuss the risk factors with their doctor.

8. Hormone Therapy after Menopause

Hormone therapy with estrogen (often combined with progesterone) has been used for many years to help relieve symptoms of menopause and prevent osteoporosis. However, some studies have shown that hormone replacement therapy after menopause increases the risk of breast cancer, the chances of dying from breast cancer, and the likelihood that the cancer may be found at a more advanced stage.

Bioidentical hormones are human-made hormones derived from plant estrogens that are chemically identical to those naturally found in people. Many integrative doctors believe these hormones are a safer way to treat the symptoms of menopause. There are also doctors who believe that *all* estrogen hormones can add fuel to the cancer. More studies need to be done.

9. Breastfeeding

Some studies suggest that breastfeeding an infant may slightly lower the risk of breast cancer, especially if it's continued for eighteen months to two years.

After participating in a whale-watching adventure, I learned that the orca whales born off the coast of British Columbia have a 50 percent survival rate due to pollution and dwindling food supply. Female orcas on average live longer than the males. Scientists believe that this is because when mother whales nurse their young, it detoxifies their bodies. Although nursing can lessen the survival rates of baby whales due to ingesting toxins, it contributes to the longevity of the mothers.

What about humans? Is it important for an expectant mother to detoxify and eat clean foods so she does not transfer chemicals to her newborn child? And will breastfeeding help a mother's body detox? Quite possibly. Today, many young mothers are committing to ridding their bodies of toxins before having children. I applaud them for that.

10. Certain Inherited Genes

Current research now indicates that only 5-10 percent of all cancer cases can be attributed to genetic defects, whereas the remaining 90-95 percent have their roots in environmental and lifestyle factors.[5]

My Paul-Like Defense

Every time I went for my annual mammogram, I read through these risk factors. I had none of them. When the nurse told me I had breast cancer, and the next week she said it was aggressive, I was devastated! My initial thought was *No way!* And then I proceeded to offer up a defense rivaling the apostle Paul's defense of himself as a true Jew (Acts 21–22). The "buts" rolled from my mouth:

But I'm not a drinker—I'm a Baptist!
But I'm not overweight! (Does my pot belly count?)
But I exercise regularly and eat healthier than most people!
But I'm not a smoker!
But I'm not sixty yet! (Just close at fifty-eight.)
But I had three children before I was thirty!
But I never used birth control pills!
But I never took estrogen hormone replacement!

But I breastfed all my babies up to two years!

But my testing showed no genetic factors!

But I'm not the kind of person who gets breast cancer!

The "buts" continued spinning around in my head. I kept picturing this obese person who could barely fit into a restaurant booth, smoking cigarettes and chomping down on a greasy burger with fries aplenty while drinking a milkshake chased down by three beers and a hot fudge sundae. And *I'm* the one who got cancer?

It made no sense. I joked with my Baptist cancer survivor friends with whom I shared a similar lifestyle and said, "Our Baptist lifestyle is not working out. Maybe it's time to start smoking, drinking, and walking on the wild side." I laughed, and that laughter helped to relieve much stress.

One day my son Harrison said, "Mom, you've always said that cancer is mainly a lifestyle disease. What do you think now?"

"I still strongly believe, as the current research suggests, that most cancers and many diseases such as Alzheimer's disease are lifestyle-related. I intend to discover what I did to contribute to this."

The Journey Begins

This was my quest: a journey to discover how I got such an aggressive cancer. CTCA ruled out genetics. So what had I done to develop a cancer that the American Cancer Society says I'm not especially at risk for? No stone would be left unturned in my quest to find out *why*.

I hate cancer and the suffering it has caused so many adults and especially children. I despise that it has taken many early from their service to our Lord. I loathe the treatments. I had hoped never to subject my body to chemotherapy.

What is chemotherapy? Cancerous cells reproduce in an uncontrollable manner, and chemotherapy drugs interfere with a cancer cell's ability to reproduce. Unfortunately, chemo is a poisonous concoction that leads to unpredictable outcomes in a person's body.

Art Rogers, an Oklahoma pastor fighting stage IV esophageal cancer, shared on his blog the four possible responses to chemotherapy according to his oncologist:

1. Chemo works, with few side effects
2. Chemo works, with severe side effects
3. Chemo doesn't work, with few side effects
4. Chemo doesn't work, with severe side effects

Everyone hopes and prays for option number one. Art, unfortunately, ended up with option four. His cancer was his "ticket to heaven." I knew others who actually died as a result of their first dose of chemotherapy. This left me to ponder, *What can I do to increase my chances of ending up with outcome number one? What can I do to help my doctor beat my cancer?* What I found makes up much of what you will read in this book.

Of course, cancer prevention is my main reason for writing this book. If only I could go back and practice what I've learned, but I can't. I can only go forward and try to prevent recurrence. I can help others prevent this nightmare and assist them in the journey. Today, many people with minimal risk factors are getting cancer. We must find the reasons. We must realize that we all live in Kansas, where twisters are a normal part of life. One can hit at any time.

I have become more convinced than ever that cancer is primarily a lifestyle-related disease, and even those with high-risk genetic factors can implement certain lifestyle modifications to change their destiny. Your genes may load the gun, but your environment pulls the trigger. The toxic soup we are all living in is overloading our immune systems.

God has created our bodies with an amazing built-in capacity to heal. Most of the time, our bodies can recover from damage caused by accidents, our own poor choices, and our lifestyle habits. My journey down the Yellow Brick Road has taught me that we serve an amazing God—the loving Creator who instructed us to care for our temples so we can serve and glorify Him (1 Corinthians 6:19–20).

Many times I have failed my God with my poor choices. But I begged His forgiveness, and you may choose to do the same.

Eight Steps to Cancer Prevention and Survival

In the next section of this book, we will examine eight steps for preventing and surviving cancer. My journey and research have clearly shown me that the same steps that help to prevent cancer can also help a person to survive the journey, prevent recurrence, and rebuild the body.

These eight steps will take you back to the basics of life—the things we've forgotten or taken for granted that impact our health daily. The first five steps are ones I've been learning for the past two decades. During my unwanted journey down the Yellow Brick Road, I have examined these five more closely and learned three additional steps to implement.

What I will share with you, my friend, are the things I wish I'd known sooner. I hope and pray that cancer never comes knocking on your door. But if it does, you'll have these steps to help you survive.

I assure you these lifestyle changes will improve your health whether you are preventing disease, surviving cancer treatments, or defending against its return. These eight steps will help your chemo to target the cancer while lessening the side effects. All of these steps will impact your immune system, which God in His infinite wisdom designed to keep you well.

My own cancer journey was a nightmare starring a wicked witch called cancer, good fairies, munchkins, lions, tigers, and bears. Two steps forward and many steps back. I desperately wanted to wake up, but I had so many lessons to learn. Let me share with you what I learned that enabled me to survive this long, but temporary nightmare.

May these lessons be a blessing for you and your loved ones in the prevention of cancer and improvement of your health. May we all find our eternal destination "over the rainbow" where cancer is feared no more. Amen.

STEP ONE:

WATER

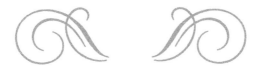

CHAPTER 2

Hydrating Your Body

But whoever drinks of the water that I will give him will never be thirsty again. The water that I will give him will become in him a spring of water welling up to eternal life.
—John 4:14 (esv)

Not long after departing Egypt, God's chosen people found themselves in the wilderness where water was scarce. They were thirsty, and they complained to Moses. So Moses cried out to the Lord, and God provided water (Exodus 17:1–6). Water is mentioned more than 600 times in the Bible, where it is acknowledged as a physical necessity and a sign of God's blessing and provision. Throughout history, wars have been fought over access to water, and every major city and civilization has been established based on proximity to water. Yet today we tend to take this life-sustaining resource for granted.

The human body needs water to live. The body can survive five to seven weeks without food, but most can last only five days without water. At least 60 percent of your body is made of water, and every living cell in your body needs it to keep functioning.

Consider the impact of water on each of your bodily systems. The circulatory system must have sufficient water to pump blood to and from the heart and deliver nutrients and oxygen to the cells. Dehydration of these cells can lead to high blood pressure, strokes, heart failure, and dementia.

The excretory system needs water to properly filter and remove toxins through the kidneys. The digestive system requires water to digest food, produce saliva, deliver nutrients through your small intestine to the bloodstream, and remove waste and toxins through your lymphatic system and colon. An insufficient supply of water to these systems leads to indigestion, peptic ulcers, constipation, kidney stones, bladder infections, kidney disease, etc.

Additionally, water is critical to the efficient function of your nervous, respiratory, and endocrine systems. Even your skeletal system requires the lubricating effects of water to protect your joints and bones.

Water has also been shown to slow the aging process, maintain memory, and improve one's attention span. In fact, water impacts every cell, tissue, organ, and system in the human body. Our blood and kidneys are 82 percent water. Our brain tissue, cells, and muscles are 75 percent water. Even our bones are 25 percent water.

This information should make hydration of your body your number one health-related goal.

The Water and Cancer Connection

Your immune and lymphatic systems can't perform their God-given purposes if your hydration is insufficient. Many researchers point to water as an important nutrient for preventing cancer. The *Journal of Clinical Oncology* has published research indicating that the more water a person drinks, the less likely he or she is to develop breast, bladder, and colon cancers.[1] Other studies show that proper hydration can reduce the risk of colon cancer by 45 percent,[2] bladder cancer by 50 percent,[3] and reduce the risk of breast cancer as well.[4]

Dr. Susan Kleiner, an assistant professor in nutrition at the University of Washington in Seattle, wrote, "New research indicates that water consumption can have an effect on the risk of urinary stone disease, and cancers of the breast, colon, and urinary tract."[5]

Simply put, without the proper intake of water, we can't move as well, think clearly or pay attention as well, nourish our cells adequately, detoxify our bodies sufficiently, or maintain our mental health. Drinking water increases the efficiency of your immune system and also helps fight depression. All of these functions help the human body to prevent cancer.

A glass of water never looked so good! (Especially when you consider that water also reduces wrinkles and the effects of aging.) Our lives depend on thousands of chemical reactions designed to take place in our beautifully and wonderfully made bodies, which are fueled by water. Ocean Robbins of the Food Revolution Network calls water "a powerful health-giving elixir."[6]

The Body Cries for Water

Dr. Fereydoon Batmanghelidj, an Iranian medical doctor who was imprisoned in his country, made water his life's work. When his fellow prisoners came to him in desperation for help, water was the only medicine he could administer from his empty black bag. Yet he found that it cured many ailments. He decided to research water rather than worry about whether he would be shot.

When he appeared before a judge, Batmanghelidj begged him, "Even if you shoot me, don't lose this information," referring to his research on water.

The judge replied, "You've made a tremendous discovery for the future," and decided to release him early.[7] Yet Batmanghelidj chose to remain in prison for the last four months of his sentence to continue treating prisoners.

After his release, he left the country and smuggled his research across the border. His work eventually led him to the University of Pennsylvania, where he continued studying the impact of water on the body. His research would prove controversial in the American medical community, gathering both criticism and acclaim among doctors while drawing the ire of the pharmaceutical industry.

"Water," he proclaimed, "is the main energy of the body especially in the brain and nervous system." He believes that a dry mouth is not the only sign of dehydration, and that nothing is utilized in our bodies without water. When patients came to him with complaints, his first response often was, "You are not sick. You are thirsty."[8]

In his bestselling book *Your Body's Many Cries for Water*, Dr.

Batmanghelidj claimed that water serves people better than drugs, saying most medical professionals do not understand the vital role of water in the human body.[9] Because every function of the body is connected to the flow of water, he stressed that water intake should be considered before warning signals are silenced with drugs. He listed the following ailments among those influenced by dehydration:

Asthma and Allergies
Diabetes
Peptic ulcers
Kidney Stones
Headaches
Heartburn
High Blood Pressure
High Cholesterol
Migraines
Lupus
Rheumatoid Pain
Joint Pain
Cancer[10] (!)

Batmanghelidj wrote that dehydration is the leading stressor of the human body. He believed that brain cell dehydration is a primary cause of Alzheimer's disease, and that cancer is a complication of chronic dehydration. At the International Conference of Cancer Researchers in 1987, he said, "Chronic dehydration produces systematic disturbances and is a primary causative factor for tumor production."

The Work of Dr. Otto Warburg

Dr. Batmanghelidj is not the only person to connect dehydration with cancer. Dr. Otto Warburg, who won the Nobel Prize in 1931 for his cancer research, believed that tumors were primarily caused by a lack of oxygen and other nutrients to the cells due to toxic accumulation and acidosis in the body.

In 1924, he concluded that cancer cells grow due to anaerobic (without oxygen) respiration and use sugar fermentation for energy, whereas healthy cells thrive in an aerobic (with oxygen) environment using protein for energy. Warburg said, "All normal cells have an absolute requirement for oxygen, but cancer cells can live without it."[11]

Since water is key to the transport of oxygen to the cells and removal of toxins from the body, chronic dehydration opens the door for cancer.

Nancy Hearn, a certified nutritional consultant, has said, "Lack of oxygenation and toxin accumulation also make the body much more vulnerable to systemic proliferation of microbes, such as certain bacteria, viruses, and fungi that are associated with cancer."[12]

How Much Water and When?

In the 1980s and '90s, soda dominated the beverage industry. According to the *Beverage Daily*, water has risen to the top of consumer preferences the past few years, with brewed teas second, and soda third. Why the change? After many doctors and nutritionists exposed the truth about the health impact of drinking sugary drinks loaded with chemicals, Americans began turning to water as their drink of choice.[13] My husband and I removed soda from our pantry more than twenty years ago because it offers no nutritional value, adds many unneeded calories, and causes a person's blood sugar to spike.

So how much water should you be drinking? Take your body weight in pounds and divide by two. That's how many ounces of water your body needs daily. For example, if you weigh 150 pounds, you need to consume seventy-five ounces of water each day under normal conditions. You may need to drink more water depending on your activity level. Some nutritionists recommend up to a gallon of water daily.

For example, if you go out for a run, visit a sauna, or just enjoy the outdoors in warm temperatures, you will need to replace what you sweat through your pores. If you feel a cold or flu coming on, you also need to increase your water intake. If you travel to higher altitudes, you must also increase water intake to raise your oxygen levels, which are decreased because the surrounding air is thinner.

Most doctors and nutritionists recommend drinking two glasses of water upon waking to replenish your water supply after sleeping. Then drink water every two hours throughout the day. Gauge what works best for you in the evening to avoid having to visit the bathroom in middle of the night.

Some people say they have trouble increasing their water intake because they don't like the taste. If that's you, the problem could be that you've trained your taste buds to crave coffee, juice, soda, etc. If so, you can also train your taste buds to desire water, a healthier choice. To help make sure I get enough water, I add stevia and garnish my drink with fresh lemon or mint making the water more enticing.

It's best not to drink a lot of water with your meals. According to Dr. Don Colbert, "It is important to limit your water to 4–8 ounces when eating. When you drink too much water with a meal, it washes out the hydrochloric acid, digestive juices, and enzymes in your stomach and intestines, which delays digestion."[14]

A good way to gauge your water input is to check the color of your urine. A well-hydrated person tends to produce colorless urine. Of course, you must also consider the color of any supplements and food you've ingested as well.

The Doctor Prescribes:

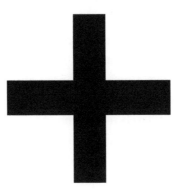

Drinking Water

Hydration is required for the proper function of your cells' metabolism. Water is absolutely necessary for protecting the cell membranes, removing cellular waste products, and ensuring that pores and receptors correctly traffic the cells' nutrients. Proper hydration also supports healthy kidney function and limits the adverse side effects of chemotherapy. Drinking a healthy amount of water is perhaps the simplest, most cost-effective step on the road to remission and prevention.

Dr. Robert L. Elliott

What Counts as Water?

The best water to drink is spring water or water that has been filtered to remove chemicals. Also, 100 percent juices, milk, and herbal teas without caffeine count as a glass of hydration. Caffeinated coffee, teas, and most soft drinks do not count as they actually force more water out of your system.

A cup of coffee contains 95–165 mg of caffeine, whereas decaffeinated coffee contains only 3–5 mg of caffeine. Most soft drinks contain 35–69 mg of caffeine in a twelve-ounce can. Sprite and ginger ale contain no caffeine and are not dehydrating drinks. However, any soft drink can contribute to high acidity levels in your body.

According to Dr. Batmanghelidj, caffeine is a drug that acts on the kidneys and causes increased urine production.[15] He also said, "The effect of caffeine on the brain is energy depletion, and if taken repeatedly, eventually exhausts the brain."[16] Caffeine is a diuretic that is, physiologically, a dehydrating agent.

Wine and beer also act as a diuretic and tend to dehydrate a person's body. When drinking, you must use moderation and replace the water lost by drinking additional water. If you want a cup of coffee in the morning or a glass of wine in the evening, you need to drink an extra glass of water soon afterward.

If traveling in a car or on a plane, make sure you are drinking ample water. Travel tends to cause dehydration. I carry a twenty-ounce glass bottle coated with protective rubber or a large Yeti cup and refill as I travel. Today, many transport hubs and hotels offer filtration refill stations.

The Benefits of Molecular Water

After the nuclear plant radiation leak at Chernobyl in 1986 and more than three million resulting cancer incidents, Dr. Igor Smirnov led a team of Russian scientists to study why some people after Chernobyl did *not* contract cancer.

The scientists found that the secret was in the unique molecular structure of the spring mineral water they had been drinking from the Caucasus Mountains. The geomagnetic field of this spring water actually hydrated their bodies' cells three times faster and more efficiently than normal, thus lessening the harmful effects of their radiation exposure. Dr. Howard Fisher, an anti-aging expert who worked with Dr. Smirnov, writes, "If you can super hydrate a cell so that it functions optimally, that cell can basically take on almost anything."[17]

In 2000, Dr. Smirnov received a patent on replicating this water, which is now called Molecular Resonance Effect Technology (MRET) activated water. MRET products are now available through www.giawellness.com.

Research done at Kiev State University showed that mice that drank MRET water before being injected with cancer cells lived 70 percent longer, and the inhibition of cancer cells was 52 percent better, than a control group that drank regular water. There is evidence to suggest that hydration of the cell is a key to battling all kinds of diseases, including cancer.[18]

Dr. Mu Shik Jhon has done extensive research on a similar type of molecular water called "hexagonal water." His hexagonal water is also thought to provide greater energy, rapid hydration, better nutrient absorption, and enhanced immune function. Filters for making this water are sold at www.nikken.com.

Pairing Plants with Water

Anthropologist Gina Bria believes that hydration is more than drinking just water. To her, water is not always blue. It's also green. Her research on hydration gathered from desert communities indicated that desert people use a combination of plants and water to hydrate. She describes plants as "gifts of nature packed with nutrients and fiber to enhance absorption."[19] Since plants are 80-90 percent water, she advocates pairing plants and water to increase hydration in cells.

Bria promotes smoothies as providing more hydration than juicing due to their fiber content. She believes that people now need more hydration than previously because we are living mainly indoors and using dehydrating medications.

She is also an advocate of daily exercise. Bria says, "Movement is key to how your body transfers moisture to all of your body tissue."[20] We will learn more about the role of exercise in treating and preventing disease in chapter 4.

Hydration as a First Remedy

For anyone wanting to avoid cancer, water is one of the most important and cheapest sources of prevention. The simplest and most remarkable remedy for almost any ailment begins with a nutrient that God created on the very first day. Pure H_2O. Water.

Whether you are suffering from a headache, constipation, aching bones, kidney stones, heartburn, attention deficit, brain fog, seizures or other malady, begin treatment by drinking more water. Then pursue other options.

The need for hydration was made clear to me when one of my sons was admitted to the emergency room with excruciating pain from a kidney stone. The first words from the doctor's mouth were, "Have you been hydrating?" My son had just spent a weekend on a Young Life trip. He was so busy having a great time, he forgot to drink water. A painful lesson learned.

My family learned another lesson about hydration when our young Welsh corgi, Reggie, began having seizures. We decided to forgo the medication and increase his water intake and exercise. The seizures soon subsided. Reggie's vet said, "It's amazing what hydration and exercise can do for the brain." It's a lesson I never forgot.

The key role of water in the human body can be dramatically seen in the final days of life. When a dying person can no longer take in water, each system of the body begins to shut down one at a time, resulting in death due to dehydration of cells. Unfortunately, I've witnessed this process twice when my parents passed.

Water and the Cancer Journey

You must have a plan to properly hydrate your body during cancer treatments. When I was undergoing chemotherapy, my nutritionist advised me to increase my water intake by adding an *additional* three to four eight-ounce glasses of water two days before chemo, during chemo, and two days afterward. Kalli Castille, a nutritionist at CTCA, says, "Good hydration helps flush toxins out of the body and reduce potential side effects of treatment, such as nausea, constipation and fatigue."[21]

When my chemo nurses saw me coming, they knew to stock water bottles at my station. Of course, this required that I drag my entourage of IV tubes with me to the restroom, but the physical benefit was worth the trouble.

The primary function of the body's lymphatic system is to take out the trash. After chemotherapy, the body has a lot of trash (toxins) to eliminate. Proper hydration assists the lymphatic system as well as the liver, colon, and kidneys to dispose of the trash. Constipation should not be tolerated following chemotherapy. When toxins don't move through the excretory system in a timely manner, they can be reabsorbed into the bloodstream where they continue to poison the body. Talk about toxic overload!

Prevention on a Budget

Consistent water intake not only will help in cancer prevention, but it will also lessen your chance of a heart attack or stroke. My recommendations for improving hydration as a means of disease prevention are as follows:

1. Start each day with two glasses of water, and then hydrate every two hours after. Remember, take your body weight in pounds and divide by two—that's how many ounces of water your body needs daily.
2. Drink no more than four to eight ounces of water with meals.
3. Limit carbonated and caffeinated drinks. These acidify and dehydrate the body.
4. Limit caffeinated coffee or tea to one cup and drink an additional cup of water to make up for the caffeine's dehydrating effects.
5. If you drink alcohol, drink in moderation and always replace the water you've lost due to the diuretic properties of alcohol.
6. Don't drink too much water at one time or too close to bedtime (to avoid sleep disruption).
7. Increase your water intake when exercising, sweating, or fighting an illness.
8. When health issues arise, increase your water intake first. Then seek medicinal help.

Of course, medical advice and common sense tell us to be reasonable. Too much water at one time can cause potassium and electrolyte levels to become dangerously low. Don't over saturate your body with water.

Going All Out

If you have the means, consider also taking the following steps:

1. Add a smoothie to your daily regimen to increase your hydration— and, of course, nutrition—by pairing fiber, fruits, and vegetables with water.
2. Invest in a device that transforms your home's drinking water, such as those found at giawellness.com and nikken.com.

Diving into the Deep End

When I discovered I had cancer, I was determined to regain my health. And every sign God provided pointed me back to the basics of life—those things we often take for granted but are vital for our physical well-being. Just as we need Jesus's "living water" to prevent spiritual dehydration, earthly water is absolutely critical to our physical health. One of the most important lessons I learned in my journey down the Yellow Brick Road was the role that hydration plays in helping our cells to work optimally and building our immune system.

Remember, Dorothy killed the Wicked Witch of the West with a bucket of water. Water can be a powerful nutrient in the prevention of cancer, and it is a much needed addition to any cancer prevention or treatment plan.

STEP TWO:
SLEEP

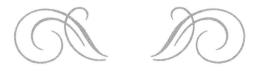

CHAPTER 3

Restoring and Rebuilding Your Body with Deep Sleep

Remember the Sabbath day, to keep it holy. Six days
you shall labor and do all your work, but the seventh
day is the Sabbath of the Lord your God. . . For in six
days the Lord made the heavens and the earth, the sea
and all that is in them, and rested the seventh day.
—Exodus 20:8–11

God is all-powerful and needs no rest, so why did He take a day off after His work of creation? In part it's because He was setting an example for humanity—He knew we would need it. God gave us the Sabbath to worship Him, thereby refreshing our bodies and souls and taking our minds off the cares and worries of this world. Keeping the Sabbath holy and preserving it as a day of rest is the third of the Ten Commandments.

The longer I live, the more I realize that God's instructions are for our protection. Modern Americans commonly have a forty-hour workweek spread over four or five days, thus allowing for one day to work around the house and another day to rest and worship.

Type A personalities like me tend to view a day of rest as a waste of time. A day with no items checked off my to-do list feels like a sin. It took me a while to understand that burning a candle on both ends is unwise.

I began to learn the value of the Sabbath as a mother of three young children, when taking a nap on Sunday after church became a necessity!

The Value of Sleep

The single most important activity we do in life is sleep. Sleep consumes about one third of our day. Some doctors are now saying that although both sleep and exercise are critical to our health, sleep may actually have the upper hand. We tend to overlook the cure to many of our modern ailments may be as close as our own pillow. And it's free!

Sleep experts recommend seven to nine hours of sleep each night. My father's own biological clock had him on his feet at 5 a.m. every morning after five hours sleep. Looking back, this was not prudent. According to Dr. Daniel Amen, a psychiatrist and brain expert, and his wife, Tana, "Adequate sleep turns on 700 health-promoting genes in the human body."[1] I, for one, don't want to miss out on those genes!

According to Dr. Russell Foster, a British sleep expert who heads the Nuffield Laboratory of Ophthalmology and the Sleep and Circadian Neuroscience Institute, 33 percent of us are not getting enough sleep. Until recently, people's circadian rhythms, or sleep/wake cycles, were regulated by the rising and setting of the sun. Because "light provides the critical input to the circadian system, synchronizing the body clock to prevailing conditions," Foster points to Thomas Edison's invention of the light bulb as the main culprit that has so disrupted our sleep patterns.[2]

In his bestselling book *The Seven Pillars of Health*, Dr. Don Colbert writes that sleep:

- Regulates the release of important growth hormones
- Slows the aging process
- Improves brain function and enables us to process information and develop memories
- Reduces cortisol and stress levels[3]

Dr. Foster adds the following important functions:

- Regulates growth and repair of our bodies

- Rids the body of protein-causing dementia (beta-amyloid is a protein fragment that is the main component in plaque)
- Develops emotional processing
- Rebuilds metabolism and replaces energy reserves
- Removes waste[4]

If you've ever thought that sleep is a waste of time, think again! Your body is performing important tasks while you're lying there dreaming away. And the deeper you sleep, the more your body works to heal itself.

Sleep Deprivation Symptoms

Far too many of us aren't getting enough sleep at night. Nodding off at your desk because you didn't get eight hours of sleep the night before is one thing, but falling asleep while driving or performing an important task can be life threatening. Some of the other serious symptoms of sleep deprivation include a slowing of thought, attention lapses, irritability, lessening of impulse control and coping abilities, memory confusion, and impaired judgment. (Is it any surprise that a sleep-deprived person can exhibit symptoms similar to those of someone who's had too much alcohol?) We're seeing an epidemic of these problems in the workplace and schools across the country.

According to Dr. Foster, long-term sleep deprivation can lead to a suppressed immune system, increasing our chances for infection, cancer, cardiovascular disease, type 2 diabetes, and mental health disorders such as depression, panic attacks, and anxiety.[5]

Loss of Sleep Affects Cognition and Memory

Dr. Michael Breus, a clinical psychologist and sleep specialist known as the Sleep Doctor, believes the human brain is affected at three different levels when we lose one night of sleep: 1) Our reaction time slows down, 2) our emotions get out of control, and 3) our thinking begins to slow down.[6]

During REM (rapid eye movement) sleep, heart rate and breathing quicken and a person can have intense, vivid dreams. As an educator, I learned that REM sleep is when our short-term memory moves to our long-term memory. This caused me to rethink my college habit of staying up all night to study for exams. Dr. Matthew Walker, professor of neuroscience and psychology at the University of California, Berkeley, says, "A lack of sleep will actually prevent your brain from making and creating new memories."[7]

Sleep Deprivation and Cancer

A lack of sleep can also greatly impair the immune system. Dr. Walker claims that after just one night of four to five hours of sleep, there is a 70 percent reduction in critical anti-cancer lymphocytes called "natural killer cells." He also believes that short sleep duration can predict a person's risk for developing numerous cancers, including bowel, prostate, and breast cancer.[8]

The apparent link between lack of sleep and cancer is so strong that, in 2007, the International Agency for Research on Cancer classified any form of nighttime shift work as a "probable carcinogen" (possible cancer-causing agent).[9] Why? Because night shifts work against the body's natural circadian rhythm. Our ability to adapt to nighttime work lessens as we age, and research continues to show a negative impact on the body.[10]

The problem intensifies when we are chronically sleep-deprived. Dr. Breus warns, "We now know that sleep affects every organ system and every disease state. The research clearly shows that a lack of sleep and exposure to disease are connected." And here's a shocker: "We also know the more sleep deprived you are, the more cancer cells multiply."[11] There's no doubt that long-term lack of sleep ages the body and inhibits its ability to perform many functions.

Natural Remedies for Sleep

Dr. Eric Zielinski, a public health researcher and essential oil expert, recommends essential oils as a natural aid in falling asleep. "Our sense of smell is directly related to the limbic brain," he says, "and smell is the quickest way to assist the body in sleeping." He recommends diffusing lavender scent at bedtime to create an environment conducive to sleeping.

My favorite natural sleep aids are Gaia Herbs Sound Sleep tea or capsules. I also like doTERRA's Serenity Oil Blend and Serenity Softgels, which include a blend of oils including lavender, ylang-ylang, vetiver, roman chamomile, and vanilla bean. You can diffuse the oil and take the softgels at the same time.

Magnesium, a mineral that also aids in sleep, performs more than 500 functions in the human body including calming the body. The best food sources for magnesium are dark leafy greens, almonds, pumpkin seeds, sesame seeds, fish, lentils, beans, avocados, and bananas. Dr. Breus recommends drinking a banana tea at night to help you fall asleep. To make this tea, cut a washed banana including the peel in half (the peel has more magnesium than the fruit) and remove the tips, place the banana in two cups of boiling water, then strain the tea. Add cinnamon and honey for flavor.[12]

You might also want to consider taking a magnesium supplement. Check with your doctor, but use prescription drugs as a last resort.

The Cortisol Slope

Dr. Alan Christianson, a naturopathic doctor in endocrinology, emphasizes the importance of the "cortisol slope" as the strongest predictor of mental and physical health. Cortisol slope is simply the difference between morning and nighttime cortisol levels, measured via saliva. Healthy bodies produce more cortisol in the morning and less at night. If you chart these levels during the day and draw a line across the results, the slope of the line should drift downward as it moves to the right.[13]

In the morning, our bodies should be high in cortisol, helping us to wake up, and then gradually drop during the day. However, some people need to reset this slope as their bodies are doing the opposite. In such cases, cortisol is low in the morning and high when it's time to sleep. Dr. Christenson advocates resetting the cortisol slope by sleeping in a cool, dark environment, implementing diet changes, getting exposure to the sun early in the day, and controlling blood sugar (which cortisol regulates and raises).[14]

Dr. Christenson cautions against drinking coffee in the afternoon, as it can inhibit cortisol reduction. In fact, most doctors recommend that you consume no caffeinated drinks after 3:00 in the afternoon.

The Doctor Prescribes:

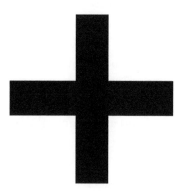

A Good Night's Sleep

Sleep and rest are vitally important for improving your stamina and protecting your immune system. For example, harmful immunosuppressive cytokines are decreased by adequate deep sleep, whereas a lack of sleep results in a sudden drop in helpful anti-cancer lymphocytes. A good night's sleep is inexpensive yet critical to your health. I recommend that you turn off your mobile phone in the hours leading up to bedtime and keep your bedroom fully dark overnight. A melatonin supplement can help induce sleepiness.

Dr. Robert L. Elliott

The Importance of Melatonin

Chris Wark, a cancer patient who beat colon cancer naturally after surgery, recommends that you sleep in total darkness because light can interfere with the production of melatonin, a hormone in your body that affects sleep. The production of melatonin in the brain is connected to time of day—it increases when it's dark and decreases when it's light. Wark says that melatonin is five times more powerful than vitamin C, and that it increases the effectiveness of lymphocytes, killer immune cells that fight off foreign invaders.[15]

My naturopathic doctor suggested a melatonin supplement to help regulate my sleep during my cancer journey. However, the body's own melatonin works best.

According to researchers at Michigan State University, "Melatonin appears to suppress the growth of breast cancer tumors."[16] In addition, a meta study of melatonin and cancer research indicated that melatonin not only reduces the side effects of chemotherapy, but also may be effective at eliminating cancer cells.[17]

The value of a good night's sleep is a valuable lesson I taught my students in public school. "Our bodies are like batteries," I reminded them. "We recharge when we sleep."

Electronic Curfew

Dr. Breus promotes getting plenty of light exposure throughout the day because sunlight improves our mood and keeps us focused. "Light exposure during the day boosts attention and alertness, improves mood and cognitive function, strengthens circadian rhythms, and can help you sleep better at night," he says.[18]

Being exposed to blue light in the evening, however, can be disastrous, as it disrupts our circadian rhythm. This disruption is thought to contribute to chronic insomnia, diabetes, heart disease, obesity, and cancer. Where do you get blue light? Electronic devices emit blue light, short-wavelength, high-energy light that interferes with the production of melatonin in the pineal gland. Exposure to blue light at night can also trick your body into thinking it's daytime. Many doctors today are recommending limiting your blue light exposure by turning off your TV, computer, iPad, and cell phone several hours before bedtime.

You can also minimize exposure to blue light before bedtime by downloading light-filtering software (e.g., Flux) on your computer and using the built-in blue light filtering settings (e.g., Apple's Night Shift) on your cell phone and iPad. Some people wear special glasses two hours before bedtime, which help to block out blue light from electronic devices.

Other doctors also recommend turning off your Wi-Fi at night. They claim that Wi-Fi can interfere with sleep for some people, and our brains and bodies need deep sleep in order to detoxify. It's a good idea not to keep your cell phone turned on or charging near where you sleep.

Sleep and the Cancer Journey

Sleep becomes even more critical on the cancer journey. Doctors cautioned me that consistent, deep sleep was necessary to help me recover from chemotherapy treatments. While up to 35 percent of adults suffer from insomnia, *59 percent* of all cancer patients suffer from sleep disturbance.[19]

Consistent, deep sleep enables the body to detox and rebuild. Therefore, I did everything possible to make sure I was getting deep sleep. This was one of the main reasons I chose not to work and retired early. I wanted to allow my body to fully recover and do the healing work God intended during sleep. If I pressured myself to get up and go to work after a sleepless night, my efforts might be in vain.

If you are a cancer patient who has been prescribed chemotherapy and sleep is a problem for you, I recommend you consider applying for temporary work disability. The cancer journey is one of sleepless nights, triggered not only by anxiety and pain, but also by the drugs and premeds you're taking. In the case of estrogen-fed breast cancer, the estrogen blockers that must be taken for a minimum of five years also contribute to insomnia.

As I mentioned, a naturopath gave me several natural sleep remedies to help regulate my sleep cycle, but a medical doctor also gave me a prescription to use when all else failed. My rule of order was simple. If not asleep by 11:00 p.m., I took a natural sleep substance. If not asleep by 1:00 a.m., I tried moving to another location to sleep. If that failed, I took the prescription sleeping pill. My goal was to get eight to ten hours of sleep each night.

Although alcohol is the most common sleep aid—at least 20 percent of American adults rely on it to help them fall asleep—drinking alcohol regularly is more likely to *interfere* with your sleep.[20]

Prevention on a Budget and In the Cancer Journey

Consistent deep sleep is not only important for your daily physical and mental health and alertness, but it may also have cancer-fighting benefits. And it's free! My recommendations for improving your sleep as a means of disease prevention and getting through the cancer journey are as follows:

1. Avoid airline red-eye specials that cause you to miss sleep.
2. When you miss sleep, make up for it the next night.
3. Avoid third-shift work if your body is feeling the impact.
4. Keep your bedroom dark and cool.
5. Minimize your light exposure one to two hours before bedtime.
6. Avoid caffeine after 3:00 p.m.
7. Keep daytime naps to thirty minutes or less.
8. Avoid eating within three hours of bedtime.
9. Avoid heavy exercise close to bedtime.
10. Use stress management techniques such as deep breathing to relax.
11. Use a white noise machine to aid sleep.
12. Avoid blue-light-emitting devices in the evening and turn off your Wi-Fi at night.
13. If unable to sleep, move to another place.
14. Use natural compounds from the plant kingdom as sleep aids.
15. Avoid using alcohol as a sleep agent.
16. Invest in the right pillow for your neck.
17. Check with your doctor about using melatonin and/or a magnesium supplement.
18. Use prescription sleep medication as a last resort.

Going All Out

If you have the financial resources, I also recommend doing the following:

1. Consider doing a sleep study to rule out other physical issues, such as sleep apnea.
2. Invest in a high-quality mattress that's right for you. Try Tempur-Pedic, Sleep Number, or an all-organic mattress such as those found at sleepingorganic.com.

Sleep. Or as the Wicked Witch of the West put it, "Slee-e-e-ep." We all need its restoring power. With a nudge from a gentle snowfall, Dorothy awakened refreshed after the poisoned poppy field rocked her into a deep sleep. Sleep is a free gift of God that unleashes daily healing as we journey down the Yellow Brick Road.

STEP THREE:

EXERCISE

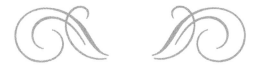

CHAPTER 4

Moving Your Body toward Optimum Health

Do you not know that your body is the temple
of the Holy Spirit who is in you, whom you have
from God, and you are not your own? For you
were bought at a price; therefore glorify God in
your body and in your spirit, which are God's.
—1 Corinthians 6:19–20

Eating alone will not keep a man well; he must also
take exercise. For food and exercise, while possessing
opposite qualities, yet work together to produce health.
—Hippocrates

The sedentary lifestyle is becoming the new smoking. God made our bodies to move during the day and to rest soundly at night. With modern innovations like cars, airplanes, and the Internet, many of us are becoming couch potatoes. Our health is paying the price, so we must actively seek ways to keep our bodies in shape.

We all know that exercise is good for us, but it is also medicine for our bodies. Just like sleep, it costs nothing to exercise and move the parts of your body. One to five pound weights are inexpensive when your goal is to build bone density. A walk around the neighborhood is a free body maintenance and strengthening technique, which can increase lung capacity, keep your bones and muscles fit, pump much needed oxygen and blood to all parts of your body, and promote weight loss. There are also many anticancer benefits to exercise.

Anticancer Benefits of Exercise

According to Dr. Leigh Erin Connealy's book *The Cancer Revolution*, the following are some of the anti-cancer benefits of exercise:

1. Boosts the immune function
2. Stimulates your lymphatic system
3. Increases oxygen and nutrient delivery to your cells and brain
4. Reduces insulin levels
5. Causes you to sweat and remove toxins from the body
6. Reduces estrogen-producing body fat
7. Reduces and helps to manage stress
8. Reduces blood-cell clumping and may thin your blood, acting as an anticoagulant
9. Relieves depression and insomnia
10. Reduces inflammation and risk of developing colorectal cancer[1]

Connealy also says, "For every thirty minutes of exercise, you neutralize twelve hours of accumulated stress in your body."[2] Managing stress is important in the cancer journey.

Dr. Daniel Amen declares, "You can add seven years to your life by taking a brisk walk 25 minutes per day." He also believes that obesity damages the brain's ability to function. Research now shows that as a person's weight goes up, the physical size of his or her brain goes down.[3] This research motivated Amen to lose thirty pounds through exercise and diet.

The stress and grief of watching my father's mental decline due to Alzheimer's disease motivated my husband and me to begin walking several miles daily. Besides alleviating stress, exercise is a great way to oxygenate the brain.

Body Weight and Cancer Risk

Being overweight is a risk factor for many types of cancer. The research clearly shows that a postmenopausal woman who carries excess body fat is more likely to develop breast cancer. This is partly related to the ability of fat tissues to increase the overall levels of estrogen in a woman's body.[4]

Dr. Robert Pendergrast describes the chain of events like this:

- The higher a woman's lifelong exposure to estrogens, the higher her risk of breast cancer.
- The higher a woman's aromatase level in tissues (an enzyme that converts other circulating steroids in the bloodstream to estrogen), the greater her estrogen levels will be.
- The greater her percent of body fat, the higher her aromatase activity.[5]

So reducing body fat without being underweight is helpful for preventing breast and other cancers.

Insulin Resistance and Exercise

According to Pendergrast, "A body that has a higher proportion of muscle mass is less likely to display insulin resistance."[6] If you exercise regularly and have toned muscles, your pancreas has to put out less insulin to maintain normal blood sugar levels. If you are not physically fit, your tissues need higher levels of insulin to maintain normal blood sugar. Pendergrast believes this strain on the pancreas is the reason many people develop diabetes as they age.

Pendergrast also points out that insulin is an anabolic hormone that promotes growth of body and tissues, but when it is present in excess, it promotes growth of body tissues in an unhealthy way. He believes this is why type 2 diabetes patients have higher rates of cancer.[7]

As someone who has tended towards type 2 diabetes since age sixteen, I use exercise to reduce my blood glucose levels. I'm just a gal who can't say no to exercise. My body requires it.

Exercise as Medication for Depression

Sweating every day not only removes toxins from the body, but also the body benefits in other ways as the lungs and heart work together during exercise—better circulation, more oxygen for the brain, strengthening of the heart, improved regulation of bodily functions, and the production of natural chemicals that help to alleviate depression, elevate mood, and enhance sleep.

Dr. Joseph Maroon, a neurosurgeon and expert in nutrition, explains why exercise is the best medicine for depression. "Exercise increases a molecule in the brain called BDNF," he says. "BDNF creates new brains cells, increases synapses between brain cells which aid memory, and enhances neuroplasticity—the brain's ability to heal itself from stress."[8]

Exercise also releases neurotransmitters such as serotonin, dopamine, and anandamide. Antidepressant drugs, which come with many unwanted side effects, release BDNFs and balance neurotransmitters, but God equipped our bodies with the ability to enhance mood through activity. Exercise is my "happy pill," and the only side effects are beneficial.

The USDA and ACS Weigh In

The 2015–2020 USDA Dietary Guidelines for Americans mentions physical activity throughout because of its critical and complementary role in promoting good health and preventing diet-related chronic diseases.

The American Cancer Society (ACS) also advocates exercise and diet for prevention of cancer. Besides quitting smoking, they recommend the following to reduce your cancer risk:

- Get to and stay at a healthy weight throughout life.
- Be physically active on a regular basis.
- Make healthy food choices with a focus on plant-based foods.[9]

How Much Should You Exercise?

Dr. Edward Laskowski, a sports medicine expert and professor at the Mayo Clinic, recommends making physical activity a part of your lifestyle.

His specific weekly recommendations for adults include 150 minutes of moderate aerobic exercise or 75 minutes of vigorous aerobic activity. Laskowski also suggests doing strength training exercises for all major muscle groups at least twice per week. His optimum recommendation is 300 total minutes of physical activity per week.[10]

I thought I was the queen of exercise with my disciplined habit of walking several times per week. I now follow Laskowski's recommendations.

Exercise and Immune Function

Chris Wark, who overcame stage III colon cancer, maintains that exercise boosts the body's T cell production, improves the function of antioxidant enzymes, and increases the oxidation of tissue. Wark says, "When you exercise, you are sending signals to your brain to live!"[11]

Dr. Robert Lustig reports "exercise increases the mitochondria in the cell."[12] In other words, the more you move, the stronger your immune system will be!

Exercise for Lymphatic Drainage

The lymphatic system, a critical part of the body's immune system, requires movement to properly gather and remove toxins from the human body. Many of our body's systems work autonomously, but our lymphatic system requires us to cooperate and keep moving in order to function.

Wark advocates spreading out your daily exercise over three different times during the day to help keep the lymphatic system moving. Using a rebounder, jumping rope, or simply jumping up and down in your bare feet will ensure that your lymphatic system is activated three times a day.

I have no doubt that exercise played a key role in my own recovery and the rebuilding of my body. From the time I was first diagnosed, I took long walks in our neighborhood to deal with the weight of stress that burdened my heart as I struggled with my dilemma. Walking briskly also helped with my bouts of depression and anxiety. In my experience, our bodies thrive when we move.

Recent COSA Position on Cancer and Exercise

The Clinical Oncology Society of Australia's (COSA) position after years of research into exercise and cancer has sent shockwaves throughout the cancer treatment community. At one time, cancer patients were counseled to limit their physical activity. But COSA now recommends, "exercise be embedded as a part of standard treatment in cancer care and viewed as an adjunct therapy to counteract the adverse effects of cancer and its treatments."[13]

Associate Professor Prue Cormie of COSA says the position paper, which has been endorsed by twenty-five health organizations, is based on indisputable evidence. She says, "If the effects of exercise could be encapsulated in a pill, it would be prescribed to every cancer patient worldwide and viewed as a major breakthrough in cancer treatment."[14]

Exercise Promotes Healing after Surgery

Immediately after my first surgery, I had more tubes and monitors attached to my body than I knew what to do with. I was told that the catheter could be removed the next morning if I were able to walk four rounds of the floor where I was hospitalized.

That was my motivation. The COSA research had not yet been published. But, after a long but bearable night, I hit the red button to summon a nurse. "Let's go," I said. "I'm ready to eject this catheter!"

It was me and my entourage—a catheter, several draining tubes attached to my breast, one heart monitor, and a disconnected oxygen mask. I made it around one time. It felt good to move, so I did it the second time with no assistance. Followed by a third and fourth.

"How many to a mile?" I asked.

"Eighteen. But I don't think you can do that!"

"Don't say *can't*."

This cancer was trying to beat me, and I was determined to fight back. While I continued walking, the nurse consulted with my surgeon to make sure it was okay for me to proceed.

"It's okay," the doctor said. "Let her continue as long as she has the energy and balance. It will only work for her good."

When I rounded the final turn of lap eighteen, there was a gathering of nurses cheering me on. I felt like Dale Earnhardt, Jr.

Before I knew it, the entire floor had taken notice, and several patients joined me to walk the hallway. I finished my tour after completing two miles.

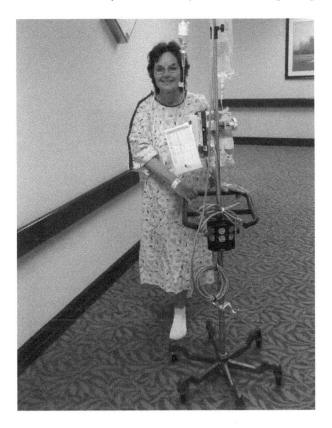

The famous two mile pole walk!

The catheter was removed soon after—a big step forward. But walking had done far more than I anticipated. The exercise had kick-started my organs, pumped anesthesia out of my body, relieved stress, lessened the threat of blood clots, sped up the draining of my breast tissue, and lifted my spirits.

When my doctor came by that afternoon to check on my progress, I received an added benefit: I went home without any attached drainage tubes. Just ask anyone who's had breast cancer surgery—that's a victory in Jesus!

The Doctor Prescribes:

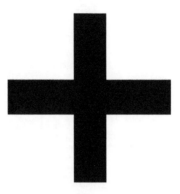

Daily Exercise

Exercise is great for improving your stamina and reducing the side effects from chemotherapy. A regular exercise regimen is also important for maintaining mitochondrial health and improving cellular respiration. Movement upgrades the expression of a transcription co-activator (PGC-1 alpha), which stimulates mitochondrial biogenesis and intracellular antioxidants. Exercise also aids in preventing depression and improving sleep.

Dr. Robert L. Elliott

Exercise Improves Mitochondrial Function

Mitochondria, known as the powerhouses of the cell, are vital to nearly every biochemical reaction and cellular process in your body. These tiny organelles inside your cells help to release the energy that's locked up in the food you eat. When functioning optimally, mitochondria increase your overall energy and slow down the aging process.

Robb Wolfe, a biochemistry researcher and lifestyle expert, says, "High-intensity exercise response upregulates recovery mechanisms within the mitochondria and our DNA." He explains that exercise corrals our cells towards health rather than dysfunction. When your mitochondria are healthy, you are healthy.[15]

Neurologist and clinical researcher Dr. Datis Kharrazian adds to this the importance of mitochondrial biogenesis, a process within the cell in which new mitochondria are self-replicated. This biogenesis improves cellular efficiency and energy. "The more active you are, the more mitochondria you make and those cells function longer."[16] After chemotherapy and radiation, I can't think of a more productive way to assist your struggling mitochondria than to exercise on a regular basis.

Benefits of Exercise during Chemotherapy

Exercise also benefitted me when undergoing chemotherapy. I made it a goal to walk one to two miles before and after each infusion. My exercise before and after treatment reduced many potential side effects. I now realize it did so much more.

Dr. Jeffrey Giguere, an outstanding oncologist with Prisma Health whom I visited for a second opinion on my chemotherapy, told me he wished all of his patients would exercise rather than lay in the bed after treatments. "Your movement is serving you well," he said.

Constipation is a common side effect of many cancer treatments. Exercise helps to keep your elimination system working to "take out the trash." If your colon doesn't move those toxins out of your body in time, they are reabsorbed into your system, and you don't want that to happen. When needed, I took MiraLAX, increased water intake, and used enemas to clear my bowels.

I've since learned that exercise actually helped the chemotherapy drugs to target my cancer as well as moving toxins out of my system. When you're undergoing chemotherapy, you want your body working at optimum levels. Keep moving and you help your doctor increase your chances of survival.

Exercise Replaces Many Medications

Research indicates that cancer patients who commit to an exercise regime after diagnosis tend to live longer and have a lower cancer recurrence rate than those who don't.[17] They also tend to use fewer medications.

With an estrogen-fed cancer, pills such as Arimidex—given for a minimum of five years to prevent the conversion of steroids into estrogen—wreak havoc on one's body. Many women taking these medications struggle with insomnia, depression, brain fog, weakness, hot flashes, bone and joint pain, and loss of bone density. For these reasons, some women refuse to take the pills. In light of the many side effects of hormone therapy, there's no better time to commit to an exercise routine, including weight-bearing exercises.

Many patients resort to sleeping pills, depression medication, painkillers, and bone shot/pills to compensate for the side effects of hormone therapy. But I recommend that women first implement exercise to help them sleep, reduce pain, elevate mood, think clearly, and prevent osteoporosis. *Then*, if necessary, use medication.

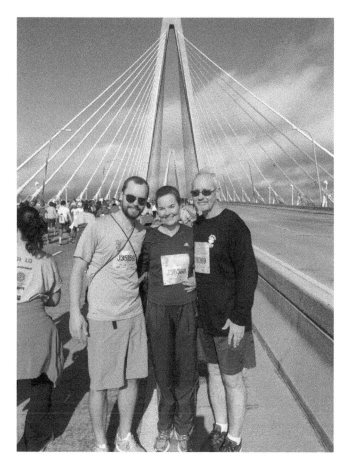

Alton, Harrison and I completing the Cooper River
10 K Run during chemo treatments.

Exercise and Preventing Osteoporosis

I received both good news and bad news after being on Arimidex for six months. The bone density in my hips had actually *increased* due to my weight-bearing exercises. Unfortunately, my spine was on the brink of osteoporosis.

I was determined to improve my spine without additional medication, so I dug further. My research led me to yoga—specifically those exercises that would help to rebuild the osteoblasts in my spine.

Osteoblasts, which are bone-making cells, secrete collagen,

proteoglycans, and glycoproteins that form a woven matrix, which attracts calcium and phosphates to form a thin lining around the bones.[18] Bone mass is maintained between the activity of osteoblasts that form bone and other cells, called osteoclasts, that break it down.[19]

Initially, I was skeptical of yoga due to its ties to Eastern mysticism. I soon realized, however, that meditation and attention during my yoga exercises could be centered on my Christian faith. I was able to meditate on Bible verses with Christian music playing in the background.

Yoga is not only good for bone density, but it also improves mood, relieves stress, increases strength and flexibility, and oxygenates the body, which promotes healing. Dr. Loren Fishman, a recognized physical and rehabilitative physician who teaches at Columbia University, is an expert on the benefits of yoga. His book *Healing Yoga* provides convincing evidence that yoga can help some patients avoid back surgeries, relieve insomnia, and build bone density.[20]

Fishman also believes that yoga exerts a positive influence on arthritic joints. Yoga's extreme positions circulate joint fluid to the very corners of the joint, where arthritis often begins and flourishes.[21] He attributes this to Wolff's law, which states that a bone will adapt to the loads under which it is placed. Fishman says, "When bone cells get stimulated through being compressed or twisted or elongated, they produce more bone mass until that bone gets strong enough to resist the pressure." Fishman says, "Like weight training, yoga works by stressing the bone. Yoga stimulates the bone with isometric contraction at almost every conceivable angle for long periods of time."[22]

Other fitness options include joining a health club where a trainer can assist you in building strength through weight-bearing exercises. You might also consider equipping your home with fitness equipment such as a Stairmaster, treadmill, or stationary cycle. But joining a club or exercise groups adds the element of peer pressure to help you carry out your goals.

I purchased a vibration platform, which I stand on ten minutes in the morning and evening to help build bone density and stimulate my lymphatic system. The original Power Plate was designed to help Russian cosmonauts rebuild the bone density lost while living without gravity in space. You can also use a $20 stability ball or trampoline to increase bone density.

However you approach the problem, cancer patients absolutely must avoid osteoporosis. I was determined to fight back in this arena. I had been knocked down, but I was ready to get back up and fight. My next bone density scans revealed improvement.

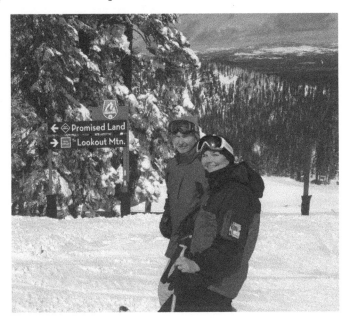

Still bound for the Promised Land with spirits high and lifted up.

Prevention on a Budget

You don't have to break the bank to exercise. It costs little to nothing to move the parts of your body. Here are my recommendations for using exercise as a means of disease prevention:

1. Walk briskly or do moderate aerobic exercise at least three to five days a week.
2. Do a fifteen-minute strength training routine for all major muscles twice a week.

In the Cancer Journey

If you or a loved one are currently battling cancer, my recommendations in addition to those above are:

1. Stimulate your immune system by exercising three times a day.
2. Add yoga or Pilates to your routine to prevent declining bone density.
3. Move as soon as you are able or permitted after surgery.
4. Walk one to two miles before and after chemotherapy, if possible.
5. Use exercise to relieve stress and anxiety and to elevate mood.

Going All Out

If you have the financial means, I recommend doing the following to help you meet your fitness goals:

1. Join a health club and hire a fitness trainer.
2. Attend yoga, Pilates, and/or exercise classes to develop a regular routine.
3. Buy exercise equipment for home use to meet your specific needs.
4. If bone density is an issue, purchase and use a vibration platform, stability ball, or trampoline.

Move It or Lose It

Ah, the benefits of exercise. The evidence is clear that physical activity is important for strengthening bones, regulating body systems, and enhancing the immune system. It's common knowledge that many lifestyle diseases such as cancer, high blood pressure, and Alzheimer's disease may be prevented with daily exercise.

"I can't afford to exercise" is no excuse. You can't afford not to. A sedentary lifestyle clearly is a precursor to numerous health problems. Like hydration and sleep, it's mostly free. The research clearly shows that regular exercise turns on thousands of genes that change your gene expressions in healthy ways.[23]

When one is on a cancer journey, physical exercise and movement cannot be ignored just because you don't feel well. My best advice is to keep moving. Do what you can when you can. Jack LaLanne, the Godfather of Fitness himself, admitted he didn't like to exercise. It's not always fun, but don't use this as an excuse.

Dorothy kept moving toward the Emerald City, and so should we. Movement allows us to glorify God as we care for our bodies.

STEP FOUR:

NUTRITION

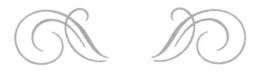

CHAPTER 5

Food as Powerful Medicine

Let food be thy medicine, and medicine be thy food.
—Hippocrates

The standard American diet is fertilizer for cancer.
—Dr. Patrick Quillin

Everything in excess is opposed by nature.
—Hippocrates

I've not always used food as medicine. In fact, my title in high school could have been Junk Food Queen. Following the typical Standard American Diet (SAD), I was addicted to sweets, high carbs, fats, and soft drinks. I was living as though tomorrow was promised to me no matter what I consumed.

Lesson One

My perspective changed overnight when I was diagnosed with severe reactive hypoglycemia. I cried buckets of Oreos when I realized my days of donuts, cheesecake, ice cream, sweet tea, Quarter Pounders with Cheese, and French fries were over.

I had been struggling to lift my head off my desk in high school until a doctor advised me to change my diet. He warned me that if I did not turn things around, I was headed for type 2 diabetes. When he told me it might not be advisable for me to carry children in the future, he had my full attention.

He referred me to a nutritionist, and she balanced my diet, severely reduced my sugar intake, and eliminated all caffeine. I had been drinking an average of four Diet Cokes and four glasses of tea daily. Along with milkshakes, those were my drinks of choice. I learned that caffeine and high carbs elevated my blood sugar and two hours later were causing my blood sugar to crash. Blood sugar must be maintained between specific levels for the immune system and body to function optimally.

The nutritionist made a believer out of me when, just two months later, my blood sugar levels had returned to normal. I felt great. My low blood sugar had been robbing me of energy for years and plagued me with throbbing headaches. This was my first lesson in using food as medicine. But my back had to be against the wall for me to make changes to my diet. Sadly, this is true for most of us.

Lesson Two

My second lesson in food as medicine was during my father's journey with Alzheimer's disease (AD). The pain of his diagnosis and eight-year decline sent me on a quest to discover what could cause such a horrible disease. I found my answer in prevention.

Attending a medical research conference on Cancer and Alzheimer's disease in Charleston, SC, in 2002, I learned that medical researchers were far from finding a cure for AD. They were recommending prevention as the only means of avoiding the illness. A doctor flashed pictures of fruits and vegetables on a screen and referred to them as the phytochemicals and antioxidants that are missing from our diets.

My research took me to a renowned neurologist, Dr. Vincent Fortanasce, a professor at the University of Southern California who had lost his own dad to this dreadful disease. He had come to realize that all of his Alzheimer's patients had several lifestyle characteristics in common: 1) poor quality of sleep; 2) continual high alert and stress; 3) a diet low in nutrients; and 4) a sedentary lifestyle.[1] These traits also described my father, Harry Dent, Sr., and his workaholic days serving three presidents in the White House.

Fortanasce's recommendations for preventing Alzheimer's included 1) aerobic exercise five times each week; 2) hydration; 3) seven to eight hours of sleep per night; 4) a diet high in legumes, nuts, seeds, fish, vegetables, and fruits (especially blueberries); 5) keeping the brain active; 6) regular meditation (or prayer); and 7) social interaction.[2]

From that day, my husband and I increased our intake of fruits and vegetables to five servings per day and added blueberries to our diet. These delicious natural delicacies protect the immune system.

Lesson Three

My third lesson in food as medicine came when my husband was diagnosed with prostate cancer in April 2004. While meeting with Dr. Patrick Walsh, one of the top urology surgeons at Johns Hopkins, I asked, "What caused this?" After all, my husband had been the picture of health.

I'll never forget his response. "The American diet is crap," Dr. Walsh replied. "If we don't realize it soon, there won't be a man left who doesn't have this cancer." His partner, Dr. Ballentine Carter, gave my husband eight months to see if he could get his elevated PSA count down through diet to avoid surgery.

We sought a second opinion from Dr. Fray Marshall at the Emory Department of Urology. Known for his laparoscopic surgery to remove the prostate, he also felt Alton had a chance to reverse the cancer with dietary changes. His office lobby was filled with prints of luscious fruits and vegetables. They were preaching a message to us.

Using food as medicine, my husband's elevated PSA dropped miraculously over time from 19 to 1. Our doctors were thrilled until Alton was attacked by a swarm of yellow jackets, and his PSA jumped back up to 10. At this time, the doctors advised us to remove his prostate. With Marshall and Carter booked months in advance, I found a highly skilled laparoscopic surgeon at Northside Hospital in Atlanta.

Dr. Scott Miller's waiting list was three months long. Providentially, his nurse let my husband in when another patient cancelled. Five days after meeting with Dr. Miller, we returned for surgery. The doctor told me the surgery was successful but the hardest he'd ever done. "It was the scar tissue caused by an infection your husband got from the biopsy," he said.

It was an ordeal, but with our backs to the wall again, we decreased our junk food and increased our fruits and vegetables to seven servings per day.

The Final Lesson

I thought we'd changed enough, but I had more to learn. And that came through my breast cancer journey. Why must I always learn things the hard way?

My journey to Cancer Treatment Centers of America in Illinois for a second opinion turned out to be one of the best decisions in my life. CTCA combines the best of conventional medicine with integrative medicine, meaning plant-based medicine and diet would be part of my treatment. All meals were provided by CTCA for their patients and caregivers. I was impressed with the array of salads, entrees, and drinks—all on the healthy, organic side. Lunch at CTCA was quite delicious. Fresh fruit and vegetables abounded like a modern-day Garden of Eden.

My diet had gradually become healthier. However, I did not yet understand the significance of eating organic foods. I'd heard that some foods contained more chemicals than others, but I assumed my body was able to handle them. Still, I knew something needed to change. After all, this healthy girl had cancer. Every illness has a cause—no scientist would deny that.

Dr. Daniel Amen says, "Your food is either your medicine or your poison." This hard-headed woman is finally now treating her food as medicine. My fruit and vegetable intake is now up to ten to thirteen servings per day, which is the amount recommended by the 2015 USDA guidelines.

Why Fruits and Vegetables Are Needed

In 2005, the USDA revised the food pyramid to include more whole foods, less fat, and more fruits and vegetables. Why the change? Rates of chronic disease in the U.S. had risen significantly due in part to changes in diet and lifestyle behaviors. The World Health Organization (WHO) had determined that poor diet and physical inactivity were primary contributors to the leading causes of death and disability in the world.

About half of American adults currently have one or more preventable chronic diseases. Many are related to poor eating habits, which include eating foods high in sugar and refined carbohydrates, high in saturated fats and trans fats, high in chemical additives and preservatives, high in protein, and low in fresh fruits and vegetables. These preventable diseases include heart disease, high blood pressure, type 2 diabetes, poor bone health, and some cancers. In addition, nearly two-thirds of adults and nearly one-third of children and youth are overweight or obese.[3]

In 2013, former First Lady Michelle Obama and the USDA announced a new nutrition icon called My Plate as a part of an ongoing campaign against obesity. (Obesity is a risk factor for type 2 diabetes, cancer, and nearly every chronic lifestyle disease.) My Plate gave Americans a simpler way of looking at balancing their diet. According to the USDA, half of your plate should contain fruits and vegetables—yes, I said HALF— and hopefully fresh. The other half of the plate is divided between one-third protein and two-thirds whole grains. A small circle above the plate represents a serving of dairy, such as yogurt or a glass of milk. For the first time, the USDA is recommending eating a more plant-based diet and using healthy oils sparingly.[4]

This is a dramatic change from the food pyramid of 1992, which listed grains (including white flour) as the primary food group occupying the most servings. The changes reflect what many nutritionists and doctors are finding contributes to good health.

Dr. Joseph Mercola, a well-known integrative and osteopathic physician, has applauded this approach but recommends that people with tendencies toward type 2 diabetes limit their fructose intake to 15 grams per day. I am definitely one of those people.

An Inverted Food Pyramid

Dr. William Sears, a medical consultant for *Baby Talk* and *Parenting* magazines, is widely quoted as saying that he believes over 70 percent of disease is preventable through good nutrition. Dr. David Katz, director of the Yale University Prevention Research Center, says, "Children are being more harmed by poor diet than by exposure to alcohol, drugs and tobacco combined. Due to poor diet, this generation of children has a shorter life expectancy than their parents."[5]

This is shocking to hear, but as one who has worked on the front lines of education for thirty-two years, I've witnessed this trend firsthand. We have literally turned the recommended pyramid of the food groups upside down. We think because we're Americans or, worse, Christians, we don't have to follow common sense in our eating habits. We've wandered so far from the Garden of Eden.

Our love of junk food and highly processed food has made carbohydrates and fats the foundation of our diet. Research indicates that the average American eats up to three fruits and vegetables each day, but it also shows that one-quarter of all vegetables consumed are French fries! French fries are a deep-fried starch that have none of the benefits of green vegetables.

In addition, Americans eat too many trans fats and saturated fats (the wrong kinds of fats), too much protein (which has adverse consequences unless you're building muscle mass), too many carbohydrates such as breads and cereals, and not enough of the most important nutrients God gifted us in nature in the form of fruits and vegetables.

Back to the Garden of Eden

Why are fruits and vegetables so important for our bodies?

> And God said, "See, I have given you every herb that yields seed which is on the face of all the earth, and every tree whose fruit yields seed; to you it shall be for food. Also, to every beast of the earth, to every bird of the air, and to everything that creeps on the earth, in which there is life, I have given every green herb for food"; and it was so. (Genesis 1:29–30)

Because God said so! In this passage, God is telling us what He created for us to eat. Did He say French fries, corn chips, and Taco Bell? No! He made seed-bearing plants and leaves to provide our required nutrients, and indeed science has shown that fruits and vegetables can actually supply all of our nutritional needs, including protein.

What else does the Bible say about fruits and vegetables?

> Along the bank of the river, on this side and that, will grow all kinds of trees used for food; their leaves will not wither, and their fruit will not fail. They will bear fruit every month, because their water flows from the sanctuary. Their fruit will be for food, and their leaves for medicine. (Ezekiel 47:12)

> In the middle of its street, and on either side of the river, was the tree of life, which bore twelve fruits, each tree yielding its fruit every month. The leaves of the tree were for the healing of the nations. (Revelation 22:2)

In the first passage, God shows the prophet Ezekiel a picture of the New Jerusalem where fruits and vegetables will grow continually in the afterlife. These trees will bear fruit every month, and their leaves will be used as medicine. In the second passage, the apostle John also sees a vision of the new earth. The leaves of fruits, vegetables, and herbs have been used as medicine for thousands of years, including biblical times and the days of Hippocrates, the father of medicine, in the fifth century BC.

Only in the last fifty years or so have we drifted from plant-based medicine to synthetic medicines. Yes, conventional medicines can save lives, but these come with side effects—just pay attention to any drug commercial or read the literature that comes with your prescriptions—whereas plant-based medicines generally have little or no side effects.

God gave us fruits and vegetables to nourish our bodies and provide for our healing. Let's look at some of the miraculous nutrients and compounds found in these foods.

The Power of Fruits and Vegetables

Fruits and vegetables contain fiber, vitamins, minerals, phytochemicals, antioxidants, and other compounds that help to fight disease. They can also contain carbohydrates, protein, and healthy fats.

Let's begin with fiber. Fiber regulates bodily functions in the digestive system. Fats and toxins attach to fiber, and the bulk of fiber moves waste through your colon to the exit door, thus taking out the body's trash. When a person is constipated, doctors advise increasing water and fiber intake. Fiber also reduces the risk of cancer, heart attacks, and strokes and helps to lower cholesterol. For estrogen-fed cancers, diets high in fiber seem to reduce estrogen levels and promote weight loss, thereby reducing the risk of breast cancer.

Fiber also helps to balance the immune system, reduce inflammation, create neurotransmitters, feed your gut bacteria, slow down the rate glucose is absorbed, lower triglycerides, eliminate waste and toxins from the bowel, and is an essential nutrient that seals the gut lining. The average woman needs twenty-seven grams of fiber daily but is getting only fifteen to seventeen grams. The average man needs thirty-seven grams but is getting only about twenty-one grams.

Vitamins and minerals are needed to regulate the body's many processes and chemical reactions that occur daily. Deficiencies result in the body not working up to par. Vitamins and minerals can be taken by mouth, but they should come from whole food sources, not from a lab where they are synthetically produced. A well-rounded diet of fruits and vegetables in a variety of colors can supply all the vitamins and minerals we need, although some integrative doctors are recommending a whole-food supplement due to soil depletion.

Phytochemicals and antioxidants are "magic bullets" for our bodies. The colors in fruits and vegetables are the "phytos," which help to fight disease and cancer. There are more than 25,000 phytonutrients found in our plant food, which travel to the cellular level and can actually change our genetic expression. Dr. Ben Lynch suggests in his book *Dirty Genes* that we can clean up our defective genes with lifestyle changes that include the consumption of more fruits and vegetables.[6]

The antioxidants in fruits and vegetables absorb free radicals before they damage our bodies and are therefore important in building the immune system. Sometimes the cells in the body's immune system purposefully create free radicals to neutralize viruses and bacteria, but environmental factors—including pollution, radiation, cigarette smoke, and herbicides—are spawning dangerous levels of free radicals that attack the body.

If these free radicals are not neutralized, the result can be cancer, Alzheimer's, and a host of other diseases. As we age, our bodies' ability to deal with outside toxins declines. Meanwhile, an increasing number of toxins are being introduced into our world at a time when people are living longer. So what can we do? Eat more fruits and vegetables.

Dr. Don Colbert lists several benefits of adding to your diet phytonutrients, plant-derived nutrients that can do the following for you:

- Prevent and fight tumors and cancer
- Lower your cholesterol
- Increase immune function
- Fight viruses
- Stimulate detoxification enzymes
- Block the production of cancer-causing compounds
- Protect your DNA from damage[7]

For the last forty years, naturopathic doctors and nutritionists have been sounding the alarm, touting fruits and vegetables as a key to restoring and maintaining good health. It's only recently that the American Cancer Society (ACS) has begun maintaining that eighty percent of cancer can be prevented through positive lifestyle behaviors. They are now promoting "increasing and eating a variety of fruits and vegetables because they contain important vitamins, minerals, phytochemicals, and antioxidants."[8]

There are now hundreds of studies correlating the consumption of fruits and vegetables with cancer prevention.[9] The ACS is now joined by the USDA, the Surgeon General, the National Cancer Institute, and the U.S. Department of Health and Human Services in recommending increasing the amount of fruits and vegetables in our diets.

In an advertisement posted at a PGA Golf Tournament, MD Anderson, the leading cancer center in the US, encouraged moving towards a more plant-based diet to reduce cancer risk by 40 percent.

The Research of Dr. William Li

There are other studies suggesting that cancer patients who eat more fruits and vegetables actually live longer![10] Harvard graduate, medical researcher and doctor William Li is now promoting plant-based food as the basis for an anticancer diet. He believes we can eat to starve cancer by using plants as inhibitors of angiogenesis—the development of new blood cells that can fuel cancer.

"Angiogenesis is a hallmark of cancer," Li says. "Cancer starts out as harmless, and without a blood supply to provide nutrients, most cancers won't become dangerous." The body's ability to properly manage angiogenesis prevents blood vessels from feeding cancer.[11]

Li asked himself, "What can we add to the diet that will naturally inhibit angiogenesis?" His research foundation is now examining the fruits, vegetables, herbs, and teas that have the highest potential for preventing angiogenesis. Berries, citrus, red grapes, teas, and herbs such as turmeric and nutmeg all show great potential. Li's research indicates that the power of these plants to inhibit angiogenesis is stronger than Avastin and other pharmaceutical drugs on the market.[12]

I would like to see the ACS and other cancer foundations fund more research into nutrition, plant-based medicine, and vitamin C infusions and treating cancer as a metabolic disease. Another area that needs to be addressed is how these natural treatments can support patients undergoing cancer treatments. Some cancer treatment centers in Europe are already using botanicals and vitamin C infusions as adjuvants to chemotherapy.

In his book, *Eat to Beat Disease*, Dr. Li points out that the five defense systems in our bodies that are key pillars to our health: angiogenesis, regeneration, microbiome, DNA protection, and immunity—are all influenced by diet![13]

The Cancer-Fighting Power of Cruciferous Vegetables

I don't like the taste of broccoli sprouts, but I do love the deadly punch they can throw at cancer and other diseases. Various types of sprouts belong to the family of cruciferous vegetables, which also include Brussels sprouts, broccoli, cauliflower, cabbage, and many others. Cruciferous vegetables contain powerful nutrients, including indole-3-carbinol and sulforaphane, that may help block the growth of cancer cells[14] and possibly even kill them.[15]

The flowers of cruciferous vegetables contain two components that appear similar to the shape of a cross. The word *cruciferous* comes from the same root word as *crucify,* which means "to place one on a cross." Dr. Colbert refers to these vegetables as "cancer blasters" and says that broccoli sprouts have the highest concentration of the protective phytonutrients found in cruciferous vegetables.[16] The ACS began recommending cruciferous vegetables regularly to decrease cancer risk back in 1984![17]

President George H. W. Bush famously said, "I do not like broccoli. And I haven't liked it since I was a little kid and my mother made me eat it. And I'm president of the United States, and I'm not going to eat any more broccoli." But if you don't like one of the vegetables in this powerful cancer-fighting family, then choose the ones you do like and consume them daily. You can also take a cruciferous vegetable supplement referred to as DIM (diindolylmethane).

Sprouts grown at home in a jar are very inexpensive for the nutrients gained. I now use sprouts in my smoothies along with two cups of kale or spinach. Even my husband drinks the chocolate banana smoothie that I make in the morning, which tastes great and contains hidden sprouts and kale along with a host of other nutrients. For the "George Bushes" of this world, you can disguise the taste—just don't divulge the ingredients until *after* you see if they like it.

Other Phytonutrients

There are other phytonutrients you should incorporate into your diet. Allicin, a phytochemical with antimicrobial properties, is found in garlic and onions. Carotenoids are found in spinach, oranges, bell peppers, and carrots and function as antioxidants. Lutein, which is found in green leafy vegetables, is good for your eyesight and may help to reduce your risk of breast cancer and heart disease. Lycopene, found primarily in tomatoes, may reduce the risk of heart attacks and cancer.

It's important to eat fruits and vegetables from all the colors of the rainbow because each of them provides a different cancer-fighting agent.

PH: An Added Benefit to Fruits and Vegetables

According to Dr. David Williams, "Proper pH health balance is critical for good health, and maintaining a slightly alkaline pH is key to preventing disease." Dr. Veronique Desaulniers says, "The entire metabolic process of the human body depends on one critical factor—the pH of the plasma fluids. Through homeostasis, the body maintains a healthy pH of 7.4."[18]

When you eat a diet rich in fruits and vegetables, your pH level automatically moves from an acidic base to an alkaline base as measured by your urine or saliva on litmus strips. Unfortunately, the Standard American Diet generally puts most of us in an acidic situation, which lends itself to inflammation.

I first learned about the importance of an alkaline pH several years ago. When I first tested my urine, the reading was 5.0. It took me a while to get up to a slightly alkaline level. If your body readings are too acidic or too alkaline, your ability to absorb and break down nutrients becomes more difficult as you reach the outer limits. An alkaline pH of 7.2 is recommended for optimum health.

Research suggests that cancer cells grow and thrive in an acidic-based petri dish but die in an alkaline-based petri dish. Scientists, however, don't know if what happens in the dish will duplicate what occurs in the body. Many integrative medical doctors believe it does.

Desaulniers believes, "A low pH (acidic) creates an environment conducive to disease, and a higher pH (alkaline) promotes health. Cancer by its very nature flourishes in a very acidic environment, and the surrounding tissue that is found in cancer tumors has a very low acidic pH."[19]

Over the long term, Dr. Joshua Axe believes that acidosis in the body leads to cancer, osteoporosis, and many other diseases. He explains why calcium-rich dairy products cause some of the highest rates of osteoporosis:

> Dairy products create acidity in the body! When your blood stream becomes too acidic, it will steal calcium (a more alkaline substance) from the bones to try to balance out the pH level.[20]

He recommends eating lots of alkaline, green leafy vegetables to prevent osteoporosis. Green juices actually alkalize, oxygenate, and super-hydrate the body. That's why you see so many heath nuts juicing and consuming these powerful drinks.

Powdered green drinks are a great addition to your diet. They are alkalizing, hydrating, and add the power of fruits and vegetables to your day. I drink one daily. It's important to choose one that agrees with your taste buds, contains mainly organic ingredients, includes a variety of fruits and vegetables, and contains good probiotics.

Alkaline foods include vegetables; oils such as coconut, flax, and olive; most fruits; raw nuts; green drinks; and salmon. Acidic foods include all meats except salmon, wheat, pastas, breads, dairy products, most grains, vegetable oils, saturated fats, and most prescription medications. Drinks such as sodas, beer, and alcohol are also acidic.

Soda is simply an acidifying chemical drink that offers no nutritional benefit or hydrating value (unless there's no caffeine) to the body. It's no secret that a can of soda can be used to remove the corrosion off a car battery, clean a toilet, or remove rust from metal.

Beans: The Economic Superfood

Have you ever wondered why Mexican restaurants are so often reasonably priced? It's because inexpensive beans are among their main ingredients. According to Dr. Ann Kulze, "Beans are a nutritional powerhouse second only to vegetables in nutrients, and loaded with protein, a full spectrum of minerals, folate, and antioxidants."[21]

Journalist Dan Buettner, in a partnership with *National Geographic Magazine,* researched the five areas in the world where people live longest and identified their dietary habits. Beans were a dietary staple in Okinawa, Japan; Sardinia, Italy; Nicoya, Costa Rica; Ikaria, Greece; and among Seventh-Day Adventists in Loma Linda, California.[22]

According to Kulze, "Beans are low in calories, low in glycemic response, low in cholesterol, and protect against heart disease, breast, and colon cancers." They are easy to use in salads, soups, casseroles, dips, and as a main dish. There's simply no reason to not include a variety of inexpensive beans in your diet.

Recharging Your Immune System

According to Dr. Patrick Quillin, the former vice president of nutrition at Cancer Treatment Centers of America, protein is also an important nutrient that can't be overlooked, because it's the "backbone of the immune system." Although Americans tend to eat too much protein, patients absolutely must get sufficient amounts during the cancer journey. Cancer treatments diminish one's appetite, but Quillin says, "You can't fight a life-threatening disease while malnourished."[23]

Quillin also says, "A well-nourished cancer patient can protect against the toxic effects of chemo and radiation, thus making the cancer cells more vulnerable to the treatments."[24] He recommends eating a variety of whole foods including herbs, which are cancer-fighting agents. For those who think nutrition might interfere with or reduce the effectiveness of chemotherapy, his answer is unequivocally "No." Properly nourished cancer patients also experience less nausea and side effects from cancer treatments.[25] I can attest to that.

Come Over to the Dark Side

According to many nutritionists and physicians, dark chocolate fat and dark chocolate are actually good for you. Dr. Kulze gives five reasons why you should come over to the dark side and include this amazing treat in your diet (though limited to two ounces daily). Dark chocolate:

- Acts as a powerful antioxidant containing flavonoids
- Raises good cholesterol and lowers bad cholesterol
- Boosts blood flow and has metabolic benefits
- Provides zinc, magnesium, and fiber
- Enhances one's mood and focus[26]

Here's my recipe for a nutrient-dense smoothie that hides a multitude of healthy ingredients you might not otherwise eat and guarantees that everyone in the family will start the day right. This smoothie is also anticancer, brain boosting, detoxifying, gut and immune building, and estrogen reducing. However, if you have cancer, leave out the banana due to its higher glycemic load.

Banana Chocolate Blueberry Smoothie for Two

1 banana
¼ bar 100% cacao or ¼ cup of raw cacao
1 scoop chocolate bone broth protein (Organixx or Ancient Nutrition)
1–2 tbsp. ground flax seeds (grind daily in small coffee grinder)
1 tbsp. coconut oil or avocado (helps absorption of nutrients)
2 cups almond milk, yogurt, coconut milk, or filtered water (if reducing calories)
½ cup unsweetened coconut or milk yogurt
½ cup ice (if desired)

Hidden super foods to add in:
Small handful of broccoli sprouts or microgreens
1–2 cups spinach, kale, or other dark green leaves
½ teaspoon spirulina (careful, too much can turn the entire drink green)
1 cup frozen, organic wild blueberries

When planning our meals we need to ask, "Did God make this?" and "Will these foods nourish my body?" Jack LaLanne said, "If man made it, don't eat it."

Americans have become accustomed to a diet of excess—too much sugar, too many processed foods, and too much food with high calories and low nutrients—putting them at risk for cancer. It's vital that we stop looking at food as entertainment and start viewing our foods as nourishment and preventative medicine. We need to glorify God in our bodies by caring for them properly. He generously gave us plants for our nutrition and healing—if only we would use them.

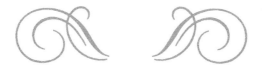

CHAPTER 6

Fats, Gluten, Dairy, and Sugar

Therefore, whether you eat or drink, or whatever
you do, do all to the glory of God.
—1 Corinthians 10:31

Now let's examine four areas of nutrition that can create problems in your body and impact your immune system. These are common foods that Americans eat and drink daily, but limiting the bad and choosing the good can make a big difference in your health and quality of life.

Good Fats, Bad Fats

Not all fats are bad. Fats are essential to your health because they support a number of your body's functions. They help the body to utilize and absorb vitamins and minerals, for example, and your brain needs good fats to coat the myelin sheaths, which coat your nerve cells and allow electrical impulses to be transmitted quickly and efficiently. But as the My Plate graphic suggests, fat intake should be limited.

One of the problems with the Standard American Diet (SAD) is that we consume too many of the bad fats and not enough of the good fats. According to the Mayo Clinic, saturated fats and trans fats are unhealthy. Saturated fats come mainly from animal sources such as red meat, poultry, and full-fat dairy products. They raise low-density lipoprotein (LDL) cholesterol levels, which increase your risk of cardiovascular disease and type 2 diabetes. Most trans fats are made from oils through a food-processing method called partial hydrogenation and can increase unhealthy LDL cholesterol while lowering healthy high-density lipoprotein (HDL) cholesterol. This will increase your risk of developing cardiovascular disease.

The Mayo Clinic promotes monounsaturated and polyunsaturated fatty acids as the healthy fats, but even these should be used in moderation. Monounsaturated fats are found in a variety of foods including avocados, nut butters, almonds, cashews, pecans, and certain oils such as olive and canola. Research reveals that eating foods rich in monounsaturated fatty acids improves blood cholesterol levels, thereby decreasing the likelihood of heart disease while promoting healthy insulin levels and blood sugar control.

Polyunsaturated fatty acids are found mostly in plant-based foods and oils and also help to improve blood cholesterol levels and prevent type 2 diabetes. One type of polyunsaturated fats consists mainly of omega-3 fatty acids. Fish sources of omega-3 include salmon, tuna, trout, mackerel, sardines, and herring. Plant-based sources include walnut oil, eggs, avocado, and sunflower seeds.

Another type of polyunsaturated fats, omega-6 fatty acids, help maintain brain function. According to Dr. Joshua Axe, omega-6 fatty acids also stimulate skin and hair growth, provide and maintain bone health, help regulate metabolism, and benefit the reproductive system. These fatty acids can be found in pumpkin and sunflower seeds, grapeseed oil, and flax seeds and flaxseed oil.[1]

"The problem," says Axe, "is that the SAD tends to contain significantly more omega-6 than omega-3 fatty acids, particularly because omega-6 fatty acids are in many unhealthy foods, such as salad dressings, potato chips, pizza, etc." Some estimates indicate the average ratio of omega-6 fats to omega-3 fats in the Western diet is about 16:1.[2] Axe suggests that the proper ratio of omega-6 to omega-3 is about 2:1.[3] The *Journal of the National Cancer Institute* has published findings that diets high in omega-6 fats actually stimulated the growth and spread of breast cancer cells. Conversely, diets high in omega-3 fats actually suppressed breast cancer cells.[4]

Coconut Oil for Cooking and Baking

Dr. Joseph Mercola recommends coconut and grapeseed oils as the two best oils for cooking and baking at high temperatures. He does not recommend olive oil for cooking due to its chemical structure, whereby heat makes it susceptible to oxidative damage. He also cautions against cooking with polyunsaturated fats—including common vegetable oils such as corn, soy, safflower, sunflower, and canola—because they are highly susceptible to heat damage due to their double bonds.

Coconut oil, on the other hand, comprises about two-thirds medium-chain fatty acids (MCFAs), which produce a whole host of health benefits. Fifty percent of the fat content in coconut oil is a fat rarely found in nature called lauric acid. While it's true that coconut oil is a saturated fat, not all saturated fats are created equal. According to Mercola, coconut oil is "rich in lauric acid, which our body converts to monolaurin. This special agent has antibacterial, antiprotozoal, and antiviral properties. And coconut oil contains the most lauric acid of any substance on earth!"[5]

In 1981, researchers studied populations of two Polynesian islands where coconut was the chief source of caloric energy among both groups. The results, published in the *American Journal of Clinical Nutrition*, demonstrated that both populations exhibited positive vascular health.[6]

Dr. Axe also recommends coconut oil for its benefits in preventing and treating cancer, reducing inflammation and arthritis, improving memory and brain function, preventing heart disease and high blood pressure, preventing osteoporosis, boosting the immune system, and balancing hormones.[7] Of course, he had my attention at "preventing and treating" cancer. Balancing hormones is just a bonus. Coconut oil also helps to reduce the side effects of cancer treatments.[8]

Since learning about the health benefits of coconut oil, it has become my go-to oil for cooking, baking, and skin care. I've become a coconut nut! If you increase your consumption of healthy oils, cruciferous vegetables, and specific low-glycemic fruits, you can greatly diminish your risk for many types of cancer.[9]

The 2015–2020 Dietary Guidelines for Americans offers the following recommendations regarding dietary fat intake:

1. Avoid trans fats.
2. Limit saturated fats to less than 10 percent of calories per day.
3. Replace saturated fats with healthier monounsaturated and polyunsaturated fats.[10]

What's the Deal with Gluten?

We hear a lot these days about gluten. Gluten refers to the proteins found in wheat, barley, and rye. It's also added to many processed foods as a binding agent and filler. Years ago, celiac disease (an extreme sensitivity to gluten) and gluten intolerance were rare. But according to the National Institute of Diabetes, Digestive and Kidney Diseases (NIDDK), celiac disease affects one in 133 people in the U.S. Dr. Kenneth Fine, a renowned gastroenterologist, is finding that the number of people with gluten sensitivity may be greater than one in three.

You might ask, "How can that be when the Bible constantly mentions wheat as a viable food?" According to Dr. Axe, "Wheat is a highly subsidized crop. As a result, hybridization methods and genetic engineering have been used to grow wheat that is fungal-resistant, easy to harvest and process, and can produce a high yield. It is also much lower in nutrients." He goes on to say, "As processed and refined wheat products took over the U.S. markets in the 1900s, traditional methods of soaking, sprouting and souring grains in order to make them digestible and nutritious has been abandoned for a fast and convenient method of mass producing food."[11]

Gluten sensitivity causes inflammation, and long-term inflammation can lead to cancer. The easiest way to see if you are sensitive to gluten is to eliminate all gluten—all wheat, barley, and rye products, including beer—for several weeks and see if your body feels and performs better. After reducing my intake and noticing a difference, I decided to cut back on gluten in my diet.

Many restaurants and grocery stores offer options for gluten-sensitive diners. I've learned to buy whole-grain flour from Amish farmers who have not altered God's gift of wheat grain. I use brown rice flour, coconut, or almond flour when baking at home, and I buy sprouted-grain breads.

Recently, my husband and I took a Viking River Cruise from Amsterdam to Budapest. The European breads were so tasty that I ate a piece every night at dinner. I was surprised when my gut did not seem to detect what I had eaten. When I mentioned this to the chef, he replied, "We use the whole grain in its original form, which is not as high in gluten as your American-made breads." When will we learn not to mess with the designs of God and that our shortcuts ultimately cause our bodies to short-circuit?

The Problem with Dairy

I absolutely love cheese—so much so that my father called me his Poor Little Church Mouse. Unfortunately, most U.S. dairy products contain unhealthy chemicals such as antibiotics, bovine growth hormones, and pesticides. And it's right there on the carton for all to read. This discovery was hard on me.

If dairy cows are fed grains or corn instead of grass, then their products contain omega-6 fats rather than omega-3 fats. Research shows that omega-6 fats are consistently linked with cancer.[12] U.S. dairy products are banned in Europe because most of our cows have been injected with rBGH, the bovine growth hormone which some studies have linked to cancer.[13]

As a breast cancer survivor with an aggressive and estrogen-fed cancer, I've drastically decreased my intake of dairy products, and those I use are strictly organic. (After all, I'm still that church mouse who needs her cheese.) All milk-producing cows have high levels of estrogen, but "organic" on the carton indicates the product comes from cows raised without antibiotics or hormones and fed grass instead of GMO grains.

The Doctor Prescribes:

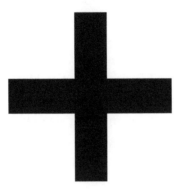

Good Food Choices

Maintaining proper nutrition is extremely important while undergoing cancer treatment. Intake of carbohydrates should be restricted whenever disease is active in the body. Consuming fewer carbohydrates decreases the glycolytic metabolism of cancer cells— the "Warburg Effect"—and promotes chemosensitivity. Cancer is a metabolic disease, and decreasing cancer cell metabolism is important. In addition, I recommend that cancer patients switch to an organic diet (see chapter 7). Also, add mushroom supplements to your daily regimen to promote lymphocyte health and activation.

Dr. Robert L. Elliott

The New Black Plague: Type 2 Diabetes

The Centers for Disease Control predicts that one in three Americans will develop type 2 diabetes, making this diagnosis the Black Plague of our day. High blood insulin levels are already correlated to Alzheimer's disease, as both high cholesterol and high blood sugar lead to problems and the formation of plaque in the brain. Sugar can also lead to a build-up of fat in muscles, leading to heart disease.

Even the co-founder of Baskin-Robbins ice cream stores, Irv Robbins, developed diabetes and had to change his diet. His son and grandson, John and Ocean Robbins, are now advocates for health and good nutrition.

Many doctors are now recommending a low glycemic index or ketogenic diet for cancer prevention. The glycemic index refers to the ability of a specific food to raise blood sugar levels. Spikes in blood sugar are a signal to the body to produce insulin, a very powerful hormone that down-regulates your blood sugar. According to Dr. Robert Pendergrast, "Prolonged elevations in insulin levels are a major risk factor for cardiovascular disease and cancers."

Pendergrast also says, "Insulin is a tumor growth promoter when its levels stay on the high side." He further suggests that type 2 diabetes patients have higher rates of cancer than the general population.[14]

Sugar Addiction

Some doctors and nutritionists refer to sugar as the new tobacco. That may sound extreme, but consider that the World Health Organization recommends people limit sugar to 5 percent of their daily caloric intake, yet one can of coke contains thirty-nine grams—almost ten teaspoons! We've got a problem when Americans on average eat twenty-two teaspoons of sugar a day (six to nine teaspoons is the maximum recommended by the American Heart Association).[15]

Did you know that a sixteen-ounce Starbucks Grande Caffè Vanilla Frappuccino contains sixty-nine grams of sugar (not to mention ninety-five milligrams of caffeine)? We are a sugar-addicted, caffeine-pumping society. According to the FDA, the average American consumes 130 pounds of sugar per person per year. This includes table sugar and high fructose corn syrup in processed foods.

Sugar, which depletes the body of calcium and other important minerals, has been linked to obesity, elevated triglycerides, heart disease, autoimmune conditions, thyroid conditions, osteoporosis, cavities, and mental health. Whatever your health problem, excess sugar will negatively amplify that condition. Dr. David Jockers gives the following five reasons one should lessen their sugar intake:

1. Sugar creates an acidic environment by over-producing lactic acid,
2. Sugar stimulates cell mitosis, boosts leptin and promotes angiogenesis,
3. Sugar drives up circulating estrogen levels,
4. Sugar blocks vitamin C uptake by white blood cells, and
5. Sugar stops normal apoptosis (death of cancer cells).[16]

In a study conducted at Connecticut College, students and a professor of psychology found that Oreo cookies are just as addictive as cocaine for lab rats. And like most humans, rats go for the middle of the Oreo first. *Dear me, am I a rat?* Their findings led Dr. Joseph Schroeder to conclude, "High fat, high sugar foods stimulate the brain in the same way that drugs do."[17]

According to Dr. Kelly Turner, "Cancer cells consume sugar (glucose) at a much faster rate than normal cells do. . . . While researchers are still not clear whether a high-sugar diet causes cancer, what we do know from Dr. Otto Warburg, who won the Nobel Prize for discovering that cancer cells get their energy and breathe differently than healthy cells do, is that once cancer cells are in your body, they consume anywhere from ten to fifty times more glucose than normal cells do."[18]

We also know that cancer cells have more insulin receptors than do normal cells.[19] Unfortunately, sugar provides a breeding ground for cancer to grow. So, if you have cancer, immediately cut all sugar and high carbohydrates from your diet!

A UCLA research team discovered that depriving cancer cells of glucose actually helps to kill cancer cells.[20] There are several low-dose chemotherapy oncologists who have been able to lower chemotherapy treatments to one-fifth to one-tenth the normal dose because they've lowered their patients' blood sugar levels.[21]

When it comes to cancer, the role of sugar is definitely an issue to explore. We've long known that the immune system is weakened and stressed when blood sugar levels are either too high or too low. According to Dr. Mark Hyman, author of *The Blood Sugar Solution* and director of the Cleveland Clinic Center for Functional Medicine, "When insulin goes up to lower blood sugar, cortisol goes up as well." And cortisol impacts the immune system by under- or overstimulating it.

So, here's my advice on sugar. Don't be like the rats. If you don't have cancer, cut back to within recommended limits. If you do have cancer, eliminate sugar and high carbohydrates from your diet and stop providing the optimum environment for cancer to thrive. By cutting sugar out of your diet, you may help starve a cancer cell.

Recommendations from the USDA

With the number of infectious diseases declining and the number of chronic lifestyle diseases on the rise, the U.S. Department of Agriculture (USDA) has revamped its recommendations. Here are their five recommendations to reduce chronic lifestyle diseases:

1. Follow a healthy eating pattern across the lifespan.
Maintain a healthy body weight; choose whole foods of fruits and vegetables, whole grains, and a variety of proteins including legumes, nuts, and seeds; eat wild as opposed to farmed seafood; and make smarter beverage choices.

2. Focus on variety, nutrient density, and amount.
Recommendations include eating half of your plate from a variety of fruits and vegetables, and the other half divided by two-thirds whole grains and one-third protein.

3. Limit calories from added sugars and saturated fats, and reduce sodium intake.

4. Shift to healthier food and beverage choices.
Too many of our calories are coming from foods and drinks that are high in calories, but low in nutrients.

5. Support healthy eating patterns for all.
As a public school employee, I've clearly seen a movement toward healthier cafeteria offerings. Still, many unhealthy foods are served in hospitals and schools.[22]

I must commend the Cancer Treatment Centers of America, who follow these guidelines and exceed them by providing whole foods that are nutrient-dense and organic. This was a Godsend for me. CTCA encouraged me to glorify God in what I ate and drank.

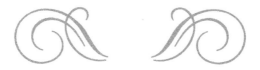

CHAPTER 7

Organics, Herbs, Oils, and Supplements

But Daniel purposed in his heart that he would not defile himself with the portion of the king's delicacies, nor with the wine which he drank; therefore he requested of the chief of the eunuchs that he might not defile himself.
—Daniel 1:8

Daniel was a man of faith devoted to God. A member of the royal family in Jerusalem, Daniel was captured as a young man and taken into captivity in Babylon where he served in the court of Nebuchadnezzar and three subsequent kings. He believed that his service and testimony to God would be impacted by his health and diet. When offered the riches of the king's food and wine, Daniel declined, insisting on a diet of seed plants and water. He believed he would fare better than those who feasted on the king's food.

This was Daniel's request:

> "Please test your servants for ten days, and let them give us vegetables to eat and water to drink. Then let our appearance be examined before you, and the appearance of the young men who eat the portion of the king's delicacies; and as you see fit, so deal with your servants."

So he consented with them in this matter, and tested them ten days. And at the end of ten days their features appeared better and fatter in flesh than all the young men who ate the portion of the king's delicacies. Thus the steward took away their portion of delicacies and the wine that they were to drink, and gave them vegetables. (Daniel 1:12–16)

There has been much discussion about why Daniel refused to eat the king's food. Was it because the Babylonians did not share Israelite dietary laws in Leviticus 11 for clean and unclean food? Was it that the meat had been sacrificed to idols? Was it that Daniel knew the king's delicacies were unhealthy? Or was it all three? Maybe Daniel had read Solomon's wisdom in Proverbs 23:1–3:

When you sit down to eat with a ruler, consider carefully what is before you; and put a knife to your throat if you are a man given to appetite. Do not desire his delicacies, for they are deceptive food.

In the King James Version, Daniel asks that he and his companions be fed "pulse," which is literally fruits and vegetables grown from seeds. It would appear that he wanted the diet prescribed in Genesis by God Himself—whole plant food that is unprocessed and unrefined. In other words, he proposed to eat what God had given Adam and Eve to eat.

We may not know the exact reasons Daniel took this stand, but we do know that Daniel and his comrades thrived. Many believe that Queen Esther also ate the same plant-based diet as part of her beauty regimen.

This is the diet I've been using to heal my body from cancer and the devastating effects of chemotherapy—unprocessed and unrefined whole, organic fruits and vegetables loaded with antioxidants and phytochemicals.

How many of us would have gladly eaten all the king's delicacies and wine if offered? Today, such delicacies are readily available at your grocery store in the form of high-caloric food and desserts loaded with trans fats and high-fructose corn syrup. Today the king of Babylon might feast on barbecued ribs, French fries dipped in ranch dressing, a chocolate fudge brownie sundae, and a Starbucks Frappuccino. We often call this "comfort food," but isn't it comforting to know that there are still foods available that will actually help *build* our immune system?

This junk food queen has eaten more than her share of the king's delicacies, and my body paid for it in many ways. Unfortunately, there are foods I've had to drastically reduce because they weaken my immune system. Trust me, the fear of my cancer returning gives me the motivation to stick to my organic, plant-based diet.

Treating the Cause, Not Just the Symptoms

According to John Robbins, author of *The Food Revolution*, "94 percent of our $3.2 trillion spent on healthcare (20 percent of our economy) is actually spent managing disease." Dr. Michael Greger says that 80 percent of chronic diseases are "lifestyle diseases." These staggering statistics point to a need to treat the cause and not just the symptoms. Daniel's diet was meant to be preventative, for when it comes to food, an ounce of prevention is truly worth a pound of cure.

Many of us show up at a doctor's office with no plans to change our lifestyle and expect our doctors to fix our symptoms with an easy surgery or pill. We are clearly a part of the problem in this country. God's wisdom is the antidote to many of our ills—we must use balance and caution in our diet.

A joint research article by the University of North Carolina and Harvard Medical School revealed that 71 percent of medical schools in this country have failed to provide the recommended minimum of twenty-five hours of nutrition-related course content.[1] If we desire to treat the cause, nutrition and lifestyle changes must be part of the treatment.

Doctors Are Waking Up

A medical intern recently told me his medical school in Greenville, South Carolina, had awakened him to a heightened awareness of the importance of nutrition. We need more medical schools moving in this direction.

We also need medical practices providing nutritional consults for their patients. Prevention should be one of our main priorities.

My eye doctor recently told me that more than 32,000 physicians have joined a network of doctors who acknowledge the connections between disease and our diet and lifestyles. The group is called the American Academy of Anti-Aging Medicine, and they educate one another as to how they can best help their patients prevent disease with lifestyle changes.

Oh, No GMOs

Before my cancer journey, I knew nothing about GMO (Genetically Modified Organisms) foods. I certainly didn't realize I was consuming them daily. How can that happen in the Land of the Free? Unfortunately, the U.S. does not require genetically modified foods to be labeled as such.

GMO ingredients are now found in more than 75 percent of foods produced in America. They began appearing on the shelves of supermarkets in 1994. The World Health Organization defines them as "organisms in which the genetic material (DNA) has been altered in such a way that does not occur naturally." These are lab-created, DNA-manipulated foods. Some people call GMO foods "God Move Over" foods. More commonly, they are known as "Frankenfoods."

So, what's the problem with these foods? According to neurosurgeon Dr. Russell Blaylock, "Some GMO crops are genetically altered to resist insects, produce higher levels of certain nutrients, and resist the toxicity of herbicides. These stronger herbicides are quite effective in killing weeds, but they leave a more toxic residue, which is passed to us when we eat it."[2]

The GMO issue got my full attention when my own test results from Great Plains Labs showed that my body was very high in herbicides and pesticides. Some scientists claim that GMO foods are harmless, that the herbicides and pesticides dissolve in the soil and do not end up in our bodies. My lab results indicated otherwise.

Blaylock admits that the full impact of GMO foods on human health is not fully known, but a study by French and Italian researchers published in the *Food and Chemical Toxicology Journal* in 2012 found death rates were five times higher among male animals fed GMO corn, and six times higher among GMO-fed females. Both male and female animals rapidly developed massive cancerous tumors.[3] Although agrochemical and agricultural biotechnology corporation Monsanto debunked these findings, many people have concerns about the amount of herbicides and pesticides that are used on crops and the impact they may have on human health. More research needs to be done.

As for me and my house, we now avoid genetically modified foods as much as possible. GMOs are found mainly among five crops: soy, sugar beets (which are refined into sugar), corn, canola, and cottonseed. These crops are used in almost all processed foods, and more crops are being added yearly.

Blaylock publishes an eye-opening brochure listing the items in our food that come from these GMO sources at www.BlaylockGMO.com.

You Are What You Eat Eats

You've heard it said that you are what you eat. But you are also what you eat eats! When you eat meat from a cow, you are also consuming what that cow has eaten. So it matters what cows and chickens eat. If you want to avoid the toxic chemicals in GMO foods, you must also avoid products derived from animals that have been fed GMO foods.

This is why grass-fed beef is in high demand these days. The demand for organic food is increasing as more and more people learn the facts. The way to avoid most of these toxic chemicals is to eat organic foods. If a fruit or vegetable is organic, the first number on its SKU label will be a 9. The *organic* label means that this crop was grown without the use of toxic pesticides, herbicides, or fertilizers. An *organic* label on meat or poultry indicates that these animals were raised on non-GMO feed and were not given hormones or antibiotics.

Why Organic?

There's no doubt organic foods can be pricier, but are they worth the extra cost? I believe they are, as do many physicians and nutritionists. Dr. Joshua Axe, who is a doctor of natural medicine, chiropractic physician and clinical nutritionist, is one of my favorite doctors to follow online. Axe gives three reasons why 100-percent-certified organic is the way to go:

1. Organic foods are more nutritious.
Organic foods have been found to contain more vitamins, minerals, enzymes, and micronutrients than conventionally grown foods.

2. Organic farmers avoid using dangerous chemicals.
Organic foods have not been exposed to the dozens of toxic chemicals that have been linked to all types of health problems. Some of these chemicals are known hormone disruptors, for example. More than 3,000 high-risk toxins are excluded by law from certified organic foods.

3. Organic foods are better for the animals and, therefore, us.
Organic foods are grown without the use of irradiation, human sludge, synthetic fertilizers, or GMOs. "Certified organic" also means the animals have not been given antibiotics or hormones, and they are fed only organic feed (not cheaper GMO feed). Keep in mind that 80 percent of the antibiotics used today are used on animals that we eat. (Any wonder why there are increasing numbers of antibiotic-resistant diseases among humans?)[4]

Herbs as Plant-Based Medicine

I occasionally used spices for flavoring my food in the past, but they are now a powerful part of my prevention-and-recovery program. Herb gardens have been used for both healing and flavoring for centuries.

Turmeric is high on the list of spices possessing both anti-inflammatory and anticancer properties. The impressive health benefits of turmeric are due to the presence of a compound called curcumin. Dr. Pendergrast says that curcumin significantly slows the growth of breast cancer cells started by exposure to pesticides. He recommends that women with breast cancer add this spice to their diet, although not during chemotherapy because it may interfere with the effectiveness of the treatment.[5]

Ginger is also a powerful anti-inflammatory root. Pendergrast is impressed with the early research on ginger and cancer prevention. "Colon and ovarian cancer have been inhibited in laboratory studies by the use of ginger and its extracts," he says. "Rosemary, another anti-inflammatory spice, has shown in animal research that it can inhibit mammary tumors induced by chemical carcinogens."[6]

Don't underestimate the benefit of both onions and garlic. A French study of 345 breast cancer patients found that increased garlic, onion, and fiber consumption were associated with a statistically significant reduction in breast cancer risk.[7]

Spirulina, a blue-green algae plant, is one of the most well-researched superfoods of our day. According to Dr. Axe, spirulina helps to detoxify heavy metals, lowers blood pressure and cholesterol, and helps to prevent cancer.[8] If harvested correctly, this is a powerful nutrient. Although the taste is unpleasant, I hide it in my smoothie daily. Check with your doctor before using it. Those with autoimmune disorders and pregnancy are not advised to use spirulina.

The Healing Power of Essential Oils

My first experience with the healing power of nature was advice given to me by a Mayan Indian in Cancun. As our tour guide, he noticed I was limping. I had a cyst on the bottom my foot, and I was scheduled for surgery in a month. He recommended that I use walnut bark tincture on the area, and so I did. Two weeks later, I joyfully showed the surgeon at my pre-op visit the miracle of my vanishing cyst. His response was, "It will be back; then we'll remove it." But it never came back!

During my cancer journey, I discovered the healing benefits of plant-based essential oils. These gifts of the earth are naturally occurring, aromatic compounds which are found in the seeds, bark, stems, roots, flowers, and other parts of plants. Use of these oils dates back to biblical times; twelve such oils, including frankincense, myrrh, oregano, and lavender, receive mention in the Bible.

Essential oils can be diffused or applied topically, and some can be ingested. As I mentioned earlier, I use Serenity Oil Blend by doTERRA to help me sleep. After chemotherapy, I used doTERRA's OnGuard Blend along with lemon oil in my morning detox drink to boost my immune system. I also used frankincense, myrrh, and sandalwood mixed with coconut oil applied topically to my breasts. Oils are now a part of my daily routine. I use them aromatically, as medicinal remedies, and as natural products to clean my home.

I did not, however, use oils on or in my body when taking chemotherapy treatments. Dr. Robert Tisserand, a well-known essential oil expert, recommends that cancer patients avoid moderate doses of essential oils one week before until one month after chemotherapy treatments. The reason is simply that some oils may protect the cells, lessen the effects, or reduce the efficacy of chemotherapy drugs.[9]

Supplements as Whole Food Medicine

If you eat a healthy, well-balanced diet, do you really need to take additional supplements? The overwhelming answer from integrative medical doctors and nutritionists is YES. Today, with our food supply so often highly processed, raised in mass production, and grown in nutrient-depleted soil, there are some essential supplements that everyone should take. Several deserve special recognition, but everyone needs to take a whole-food vitamin/mineral supplement. Zinc needs to be added if it's not already in your supplement.

Vitamin C

The power of vitamin C was clearly revealed when Paul Marik, a well-respected doctor in Norfolk, gave high-dose vitamin C infusions with steroids and thiamine as a last resort to a patient who was dying from sepsis. She survived, and Dr. Marik now regularly uses these infusions for patients in similar situations.

Vitamin C was something of a magic bullet for me. I was given these same infusions twice a week within days of my cancer diagnosis. When my chemotherapy began at CTCA, I was among the first of their patients to receive these immunity-boosting treatments twenty-four hours before each treatment to prevent possible interference. In this way, my immune system was being strengthened before the chemo knocked it down. Then in between treatments, it was built back up again. I can't begin to tell you what a difference this complementary therapy made for me.

My hope is that one day all hospitals will be using this treatment for patients undergoing chemotherapy. Oncologists should at least consider beginning vitamin C treatments once chemotherapy is over to rebuild the body's immune system. Some cancer treatment centers in Europe are using vitamin C infusions and other plant-based adjuvants such as mistletoe extract to enhance chemotherapy.

Vitamin D

All the doctors on my cancer journey recommended that I keep my vitamin D3 levels between 60 and 90 ng/ml. When I was first diagnosed with cancer, my D3 levels were at 28 ng/ml. My doctors suggested that if my levels had been higher, I might not have gotten cancer. You can ask your doctor to check your levels through a blood test when you have your yearly physical.

Dr. Daniel Amen advises his patients to maintain their levels between 70 and 100 ng/ml. Research suggests that individuals with vitamin D3 levels of 40 ng/ml or more have half the risk of getting cancer than those who had levels less than 20 ng/ml.[10] This is in addition to the benefits to the heart and emotional well-being.

Bones are also strengthened by a diet that includes plenty of green plants, sunlight (a natural source of vitamin D), and vitamin D supplements. Dr. Loren Fishman recommends 1,000 to 1,500 mg per day of calcium, unless you're over age seventy-five or have problems with circulation (then restrict your intake to 500 mg per day.)[11] Keep in mind that calcium supplements will not do you any good without vitamin D to help you absorb it.

Iodine and Selenium

Iodine is necessary for the production of the thyroid hormone and all the other hormones in the body. In fact, every cell in the body utilizes iodine. Dr. David Brownstein also believes that our increasing exposure to toxic halogens such as bromide, fluoride and chlorine derivatives have remarkably increased our need for iodine.[12] Kelp is a good source of iodine.

With hypothyroidism nearing epidemic rates, many doctors are recommending that all patients over fifty years old have their thyroid checked. Don't underestimate the importance of this small gland. It plays a major role in the metabolism, helping to regulate many body functions by steadily releasing thyroid hormones into the bloodstream. Brownstein also recommends 200 ug of selenium every day to support thyroid function and the metabolism. The human body does not produce selenium, but it can be found in meat, seafood, and nuts.

Probiotics

Dr. David Jockers promotes adding beneficial microflora to the gastrointestinal tract through the use of probiotics. Probiotics, whether obtained through fermented foods or supplements, reduce the risk of cancer by aiding with detoxification, improving apoptosis (the death of cancer cells), inhibiting tumor growth, and stimulating the immune system.[13]

Many doctors are recommending that patients include probiotic food or supplements in their daily diet. It's also important for replacing gut flora after chemotherapy destroys it.

Mushrooms

Mushrooms have tremendous nutritional value. Not only are they low in calories, but also they're a great source of fiber and protein, which is helpful when you're on a plant-based diet. Mushrooms are packed with antioxidants, B vitamins, selenium, potassium, and vitamin D.

Reishi mushrooms are particularly good for boosting the immune system, as they contain bioactive molecules that can inhibit cancer metastasis and assist in slowing the growth of tumors. There is research to support the use of reishi as an adjuvant therapy for colon, lung, prostate, and breast cancer.[14]

Maitake mushrooms also contain bioactive molecules and show promise in blocking tumor growth, especially with breast and lung cancers.[15]

EGCG and Quercetin

According to Dr. Jockers, the cancer-preventive effects of EGCG (epigallocatechin-3-gallate) have been closely studied for almost three decades. EGCG is a polyphenolic compound known for its concentration in green tea extract. It's inexpensive and induces apoptosis, supporting the destruction of cancer cells.[16]

Jockers also recommends a super antioxidant called quercetin. "High intake of quercetin in an individual's diet suppresses cancer cell proliferation, reduces oxidative damage, and inhibits the activity of a mutant gene associated with tumor growth known at P53."[17] Quercetin is found in onions, capers, blackberries, raspberries, black and green teas, dark cherries, cocoa powder, kale, apples, and herbs like sage and parsley.

Supplement Recommendations

In addition to a multivitamin/mineral supplement that meets daily requirements, here is a list of the main supplements (made from whole foods and with no added chemicals) informed doctors are recommending that cancer patients take. Always check with your doctor before beginning a supplement to ensure that it doesn't interfere with chemotherapy or treatments:

- Vitamin D3, 2,000–5,000 IUs
- Iodine
- Selenium, 200 ug per day
- Probiotics, a good strain with a variety of bacteria
- Zinc, 30–45 mg per day

- Vitamin C
- Green tea extract, curcumin, and quercetin supplement

Pantry Swap Day

After learning everything I've shared in this section of the book, I dove into my pantry, reading every label and throwing out everything that could exacerbate my condition. Some people make these changes over time, waiting until something runs out before replacing it with a better option. But I was on a mission; I had an aggressive and deadly cancer.

Here's a before-and-after inventory of my pantry and refrigerator:

Before Cancer	After Cancer
Herbs	Organic or fresh herbs (used daily)
Table salt	Sea, Celtic, or pink Himalayan salt
Seasonings	Organic herb mixes
Refined sugar	Organic sugars, used sparingly (none during cancer)
Aspartame and Splenda	Organic stevia (by SweetLeaf)
Canned food	BPA-free canned food from Earth Fare and Whole Foods
Margarine	Coconut oil or grass-fed organic butter
Commercial meats	Grass-fed organic beef (no hormones)
Chicken	Organic chicken (Coleman)
Milk and dairy	Organic dairy products (no hormones) and nut milks
Tap and bottled water	Filtered water and glass drinking bottle for transport
Sodas	Herbal teas, lemon water
Coffee	Organic coffee (in the morning only)
Vegetable oils	Extra virgin coconut, avocado, and olive oils
Roasted and salted nuts	Organic raw nuts (sprouting adds energy and nutrients)
Cheese	Organic (no hormone) cheeses and nut butters
Sweetened yogurt	Organic plain yogurt or coconut yogurt
MSG products	Homemade or store versions with no MSG
Salad dressings	Homemade dressings made with olive oil and herbs
Potato chips	Vegetable and kale chips
Tortilla chips	Organic corn chips
Rice	Organic brown rice, millet, or quinoa

Peanut butter	Raw almond and nut butters
Candy and sweets	Organic dark chocolate sweetened with stevia
Processed crackers	Gluten-free organic crackers
Wheat flour	Organic almond and/or coconut flour or Amish flour
Bacon	Uncured bacon (no nitrates) or turkey bacon, in moderation
Eggs	Organic eggs

Prevention on a Budget

The Standard American Diet (SAD) is killing this nation's people by the millions and contributing to many lifestyle diseases. As Christians, we are not exempt from taking care of our bodies. God has clearly given us instruction on this, yet we are eating the king's food as opposed to the life-giving foods provided in nature.

All of us must increase our fruit and vegetable intake if we are to remain healthy and prevent disease in the future. It's important that we eat a variety of our fruits and vegetables, raw and as close to their natural state as possible. The closer to time of picking, the more nutrients these will have. Foods should be eaten in this order: 1) fresh, 2) frozen, and 3) canned only as a last resort.

What if you don't like fruits and vegetables? Then you need to train yourself to enjoy them or hide them in a smoothie. Sure, I'd prefer to have a cheeseburger, milkshake, and fries for lunch, but my discipline allows this only on rare occasions and then only if the fries are baked and the meat is grass-fed and organic.

Once you realize the power in the food God has provided, your taste will begin to slowly change as you learn that your taste buds are not always trustworthy.

NOTE: Always let your doctor know all supplements you are taking. Some may not be able to be taken with certain chemo regimens or immunotherapies.

Here are my recommendations (Disclosure: I'm not a clinical nutritionist):

1. Start the day with a breakfast containing protein, fats, fiber, and fruit.
2. Eat the rainbow from a variety of fruits and vegetables. Include cruciferous vegetables and blueberries daily.

3. Decrease intake of processed foods, sugar, dairy, and gluten. Eat whole, fresh, live foods following My Plate recommendations.
4. Eat more nuts, seeds, and legumes for protein. Use wild-caught seafood and fish and organic, grass-fed meats.
5. Use healthy oils such as olive, avocado, and coconut oil.
6. Limit coffee to one or two cups per day and only in the morning.
7. Replace soft drinks with healthy beverages such as herbal teas, fruit juice (limited), and water with lemon.
8. Limit sodium intake to 2,300 mg per day.
9. Take a vitamin/mineral supplement, vitamin D3, kelp, and green tea extract.
10. Use fresh onions, garlic, and herbs in food preparation.

In the Cancer Journey

If you or a loved one are currently battling cancer, my recommendations in addition to those above are:

1. Consider an organic, plant-based diet until the cancer is completely gone. Your protein can come from nuts, seeds, bone broth, and legumes. You can add in organic meat, chicken, and wild-caught fish after you are cancer free. This will enable the body to concentrate on repair.
2. Eliminate foods with sugar and high carbohydrates until cancer is no longer detectable. Then keep sugar intake at low levels.
3. Eliminate dairy foods (until cancer is gone) or greatly reduce and eat organic dairy.
4. Raise your vegetables and fruits to ten to thirteen servings per day, including more vegetables than fruits and at least three servings of cruciferous vegetables.
5. Include daily fiber in your diet. This can include two tablespoons of chia or flax seeds ground daily.
6. Go gluten free to allow the body to heal. After cancer, reevaluate how your body reacts with gluten.

7. Eat prebiotic fiber from fruits and vegetables and probiotic foods such as fermented foods and yogurt. Take a probiotic supplement.
8. Ask your doctor about adding a mushroom supplement, iodine or kelp, selenium, and zinc.

Going All Out

If you have the financial means, I recommend doing the following to help you meet your nutritional goals:

1. Grow an herb garden and incorporate fresh herbs in your diet.
2. Eat mostly organic foods.
3. Add spirulina to your smoothies to enhance immune function.
4. Add a curcumin supplement daily and use fresh ginger.
5. Consider building your immune system with essential oils such as lemon and a blend of clove, cinnamon, orange, eucalyptus, and rosemary after chemotherapy.
6. Take a 1,000 mg vitamin C supplement twice daily.
7. Add DIM (diindolylmethane) and quercetin supplements.
8. Consider adding a powdered green drink daily to boost antioxidants and phytochemicals.

Disease prevention is all about perspective. When you look at your food as medicine, it changes what you put into your mouth. The compounds found in leaves, flowers, fruits, and vegetables were given by God for our health and healing. If you'll use them on a daily basis, you might never have to hear the words "You have cancer." Of course, there's no diet that can give you a 100 percent guarantee that you will never get cancer. But you must be wise in your choices.

Daniel was right about many things. What would he say about our GMO foods, sugar addiction, and the Standard American Diet? Daniel's diet included all kinds of vegetables, fruits, nuts, seeds, legumes, and herbs. Yet Daniel and his friends fared better than their contemporaries who ate the king's food. We can fare better, too. Foods with healing nutrients are found abundantly all along the Yellow Brick Road. Let us eat from God's bounty for His glory, that we may serve Him in abundant health!

STEP FIVE:

MANAGING STRESS

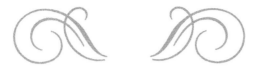

CHAPTER 8

Living Your Faith to Manage Stress and Emotions

Anxiety in the heart of man causes depression,
but a good word makes it glad.
—Proverbs 12:25

When you pass through the waters, I will be with
you; and through the rivers, they shall not overflow
you. When you walk through the fire, you shall
not be burned, nor shall the flame scorch you.
—Isaiah 43:2

Greet every difficulty and joy today with
the conviction that God has purposed it
and ordained it for this specific time.
—Dr. David Jeremiah

Stress and emotions—we all have them. How we manage these two important aspects of our lives can determine much about our overall health and well-being. In fact, dealing with negative emotions can be a key to fighting cancer. I'm grateful that the Bible gives us much-needed instruction in managing these aspects of our lives. What a comfort to know He is with us in the storm.

Numerous doctors, nutritionists, research scientists, and psychologists have emphasized the adverse effects that suppressed emotions can have on a person's physical health. Some claim the emotional impact can be up to 50 percent or more. At first, I found this notion hard to believe. However, as a counselor, I'm seeing more every day the impact our emotional life and the unconscious mind have on a person's immune system and overall health. I'm convinced that resolving emotional trauma can be a key to cancer prevention and recovery.

What's Stress Got to Do with It?

What does emotional stress have to do with your physical health? Everything! Unresolved conflict, anger, resentment, unforgiveness, grief, abandonment, and sadness all affect the body. Anything that causes your stress response to activate involves the elevation of cortisol in your body, and cortisol elevates blood sugar and estrogen levels. Sometimes, the stress response is your friend, but when it activates continuously—as with chronic, ongoing stress—it can wreak havoc on your immune system.

According to Dr. Archibald Hart, "Despite medical science's enormous strides in treating illness, the problems caused by stress are becoming more prevalent and difficult to treat. We may soon be dying less from infectious diseases and more often from the ravaging effects of too much stress—a disease we bring upon ourselves!"[1]

Each of us is equipped with a highly developed stress response system that enables a person to cope with challenging events and perceived threats. Hart warns that difficulties arise when we are living in a perpetual state of emergency. Too much stress compromises the immune system and weakens its ability to fight off disease.[2]

It's important to allow your body to heal after fight-or-flight response has been triggered and your system has been flooded with adrenaline. It's the neglect of this recovery time that leads to so many negative consequences for one's health. When stress is chronic, the immune system soon becomes depleted.

Hart also points out a connection between stress and cancer. "Stress may cause some forms of cancer to grow more rapidly because the body's ability to fight off the growth of cancer cells is dependent on its own immune system."[3] It's no secret that a high level of adrenaline caused by stress interferes with our ability to rest. We discussed earlier in the book how the sleep cycle and immune system are related, and that the body is designed to repair itself during deep sleep.

The Impact of Grief

Research for this chapter caused me to look deep within myself. Since 2000, my stress levels have been off the charts. A new job opportunity for my husband and a subsequent move forced a change of jobs and community for me. I also served as a weekend caregiver for my father due to his Alzheimer's until his passing. When the housing market tanked after September 11, 2001, we found ourselves with two house payments when the sale of our previous home fell through. And we had all three sons in college during this time!

A few years later, my husband's parents passed away, and then my mom. It was hard for me to return to work after her passing. Of course, I celebrated her entrance into heaven and her reunion with my father, but the pain of losing that final parent was at times more than I could bear. My recovery from grief was slow, but I survived. Grief requires that we pay more attention to rest, exercise, and nutrition. Taking care of my body had always been a top priority, but now my health required even more of me.

Doctors caution cancer patients to look back seven to fifteen years to determine if stress played a part in their cancer diagnosis. Over a fifteen-year period, my husband and I had served as weekend caretakers for all four parents. It's fair to say that ongoing grief and caretaking responsibilities on top of our full-time jobs kept us both in a state of high alert for many years.

It's not that we were grievers without hope. We celebrated as all four parents graduated to heaven, yet their passing weighed heavily upon our hearts. We had been blessed with wonderful parents. But, the greater the blessing, the greater the loss. Thus, I had been caught in a grief cycle for fifteen years.

Later I discovered that grief is associated with inflammation and a decrease in killer cells and white blood cells.[4] I now believe my ongoing grief and juggling a job and caregiving were both contributing factors to my cancer diagnosis. This hamster definitely needed to get off the wheel!

Research on Adverse Childhood Experiences (ACEs)

According to Dr. Niki Gratrix, "The effect of unresolved emotional trauma from childhood on health across a lifetime is possibly the most under-exposed risk factor for all major chronic health conditions in the world today."[5] Gratrix is dedicated to educating health practitioners and patients about the impact of Adverse Childhood Experiences (ACEs).

The first collaborative study on ACEs by the Centers for Disease Control and Kaiser Permanente was conducted in 1998 involving 17,500 adults. The ACEs studied included:

Separation or divorce of parents
Physical, sexual, or emotional abuse
Physical or emotional neglect
Mental illness in the family
Incarceration of a parent
Domestic violence
Substance abuse[6]

Later research added other ACEs to the list, including the death of a parent, homelessness, racism, serious childhood illness, traumatic birth, and bullying and hate abuse.

The results were staggering. Eighty percent of all adults had experienced more than one ACE. But those having four of more ACEs were four and a half times more likely to develop depression than someone who had no ACEs, more than two and a half times more likely to have a stroke, twelve times more likely to commit suicide, and *two and a half times more likely to get cancer.* Eight or more ACEs increased the risk of ischemic heart disease by three and a half times and tripled the risk of lung cancer. To top it off, a person having six or more ACEs could expect *a reduced lifespan of twenty years!*[7]

As a counselor of children for many years, I remember those students in my care who never caught a break. Some experienced painful abuse, the humiliation of homelessness, incarceration of a parent, or substance abuse by a parent. These students desperately needed continued counseling, coping mechanisms, and ongoing support. Most of all, they needed divine intervention—the grace that only God can bestow.

Both of my parents scored high on the ACE test, with my mother landing the higher score. But my mother found refuge in God. My parents did their best to make sure my siblings and I never had to experience the alcoholism, poverty, and dysfunctional life of their own childhoods. As a result, my ACE score is low. Frankly, I had a wonderful childhood. But when your childhood is traumatic, your body keeps score. If not consciously, then unconsciously. So, it's important to deal with any adverse emotions.

Biblical Instruction on Trials and Tribulations

The Bible does not skirt around this issue and clearly teaches that trials and tribulations are a normal part of life. Trials are filtered through the light of His Word and are designed to make us stronger:

> These things I have spoken to you, that in Me you may
> have peace. In the world you will have tribulation; but be
> of good cheer, I have overcome the world. (John 16:33)

Scripture tells us that God uses all things "for good to those who love God" and are "called according to His purpose" (Romans 8:28). It's not that all things are good. Some difficulties happen because of our own foolishness or disobedience, some happen at the hands of others, and some happen by chance. According to Bible teacher and pastor Dick Woodward, whatever the source of our troubles, if we meet those two conditions—we love God and are called according to His plan and purpose—God will take the bad things that happen to us and weave them into a pattern for good. Of course, that is His good and our good.

Romans 8:28 was the first verse that God used to guide and comfort me during my cancer journey. Cancer is not good. It's discouraging and horrifying. But because I am a child of God called to serve Him, He will use this horrible disease to advance His kingdom, and also use it for my good. I've heard many people say after their cancer journey, "Cancer was the best thing that ever happened to me." But how can this be?

Woodward, who suffered paralysis from the debilitating effects of multiple sclerosis, said, "God uses suffering to focus His people on spiritual and eternal values. He wants to teach us how to look up, look in, and look around."[8]

And that's what cancer did for me. It forced me to look up to God for help and guidance, to look within and examine my soul and daily habits, and to look around me for any outside influences that I needed to change. For some people, fear and a near-death experience lead to their spiritual transformation. For others, they find new purpose in life.

Ironically, my cancer journey brought my husband and me closer with a deeper love. And I've definitely found a new purpose in life!

Dealing with the Fear Factor

Cancer is a faith journey. Just the words "You have cancer" invokes a stress response. Fear is a normal part of this journey, which comes with many ups and downs. One minute you are soaring with faith, and the next minute you are trembling in fear. I can identify with the Cowardly Lion. As Christians, we are to walk by faith rather than by sight (2 Corinthians 5:7). We are not to fear, because God is always with us (Isaiah 43:1; Matthew 28:20).

As the IV was placed in my arm for my second cancer surgery, I felt confident that the surgery would be uneventful and without complications. At least, I *thought* I was confident. Then the doctor arrived and began carefully dotting my breasts with a marker to indicate precisely where he would cut, sketching a battle plan on my most intimate parts. With every stroke of his pen, droplets of perspiration appeared on my palms and brows. My mind began to whirl, and my balance grew wobbly.

"I think I'm going to faint," I said. I'd never lost consciousness before. As I started to collapse, the doctor helped me to my feet and called for support.

As it turned out, I was having a panic attack.

I was relieved to find the chaplain waiting for me in pre-op. When he prayed for me, I hung on to every word. By the time the surgical team was prepared to put me under, I was more than ready.

Yes, fear is a very real part of the cancer journey. Every time fear reared its head along the Yellow Brick Road, I felt like the Cowardly Lion. Eventually I learned that I had to face my fears head on if I was going to have the nerve to battle the cancer.

"Stay Safe" Fears and Wisdom

A moderate sense of fear can serve as a defense mechanism that helps keep us safe. For example, if I see a poisonous snake, my fears tell me to slowly back away. I call these "stay safe" fears.

In Proverbs 9:10, we are told, "The fear of the LORD is the beginning of wisdom." This fear of God is a worshipful and reverent attitude, an acknowledgment of His sovereignty, power, and preeminent position in our lives and in the universe. A healthy fear of God removes all other fears; we need only bow at His feet and worship Him.

Cancer, on the other hand, is a journey of fear—a wicked witch—that we need to lay at His feet. Yes, it's nerve-shattering waiting for the test results, knowing that life and death hang in the balance. But we must face our fears head on and ask, *What's the worst that can happen?* Christians might fear the discomfort and pain of the sickness and its treatment, but wc have no cause to fear death.

God's Word tells us that because of what Christ has done for us on the cross, we will be given all-new, disease-free, fully guaranteed bodies in which we will play and work and celebrate and worship eternally:

> For our citizenship is in heaven, from which we also eagerly wait for the Savior, the Lord Jesus Christ, who will transform our lowly body that it may be conformed to His glorious body, according to the working by which He is able even to subdue all things to Himself. (Philippians 3:20–21)

So, let's dispel any fear of death. If you are a child of God, death is a promotion—your graduation to heaven! You should eagerly anticipate the day when He finally takes you home.

His Strength in Our Weaknesses

Cancer is an arduous journey, but the Bible is clear that God's strength is made known through our weakness. When we are weak, He is strong:

> And He said to me, "My grace is sufficient for you, for
> My strength is made perfect in weakness." Therefore most
> gladly I will rather boast in my infirmities, that the power
> of Christ may rest upon me. (2 Corinthians 12:9)

I grew up in an introverted shell. Just speaking to people was excruciating for me and getting up on stage was unthinkable. I also struggled with reading and writing. When I turned over the reins of my life to Jesus Christ, things began to change. Those difficult things have since become my strengths. This is part of what God does in our lives— His strengths are made manifest in our weaknesses.

My weaknesses were front and center as I faced claustrophobic MRIs, PICC lines being inserted into my artery, five surgeries, chemotherapy, and the loss of every hair on my body. But God gave me the strength to stay the course and overcome my fears and weaknesses.

People like to say that God never gives us more than we can handle, but that isn't what the Bible teaches at all! God *often* gives us much more than we can handle so that we will turn to Him in desperate, complete dependence. His power and grace are made known in our helplessness. If we will let go of the reins and acknowledge His sovereignty in our lives, He will give us the tenacity and strength to endure—and even thrive!

The Doctor Prescribes:

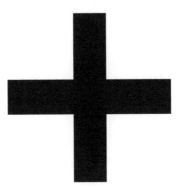

Keeping the Faith

In my experience, patients who have a strong faith and belief in God are better equipped to accept and travel the cancer journey. They tend to experience less stress and sleep better, allowing their immune systems to respond more effectively to therapy. Their willingness to surrender to God allows them to walk the cancer journey with courage, knowing that adversity leads to spiritual growth. This means that people of faith may avoid some of the anger that many cancer patients experience, thus reducing the immunosuppressive effects of stress on the body.

Dr. Robert L. Elliott

Controlling Anger

The Bible commands us not to hold our anger inside: "Do not let the sun go down while you are still angry" (Ephesians 4:26, NIV). But it also tells us not to allow our anger to get out of control: "A fool gives full vent to his anger, but a wise man quietly holds it back" (Proverbs 29:11, ESV).

Anger is the emotion that has the greatest impact on a person's heart, brain, and digestive and nervous systems. Nothing can trigger the stress response in one's body quite like uncontrolled anger. Sustained anger will cause your adrenal glands to pump out too much adrenalin and cortisol, which over time can suppress the immune system while opening the door to many diseases.

The Bible instructs us instead to control and resolve our anger. How many of us have said or done something in a rage only to regret it later? Psychologists encourage us to "Take a deep breath, count to ten, until you feel calm again." It's about self-control, waiting to think through your actions, and talking about your feelings. The truth is that your anger will hurt you more than the target of your wrath. Don't let it!

Sin, Guilt, and Confession

If you have sinned, the Lord will forgive you if you confess:

> If we confess our sins, He is faithful and just to forgive us our sins and to cleanse us from all unrighteousness. (1 John 1:9)

Guilt emerged from my cancer diagnosis when I realized that I had not taken proper care of the body God had given me. Many people told me I should not feel guilty, but the more I studied nutrition, toxins, the importance of a healthy gut, and the impact of stress on a body, the more I was certain I had fallen short.

I asked God to forgive me. I also asked Him to give me the strength to change those habits that did not benefit my body. God is always faithful to forgive when we confess with a repentant heart.

The Power of Forgiveness

Nothing has more power over our health than when we harbor resentment and unforgiveness. The world and its entertainment tell us to seek revenge when someone hurts us. (See *Gladiator*, *The Sting*, or just about any Liam Neeson movie of the past ten years.) But the Bible mentions the concept of forgiveness more than a hundred times and leaves us no wiggle room. We are commanded to forgive others as God has forgiven us:

> "For if you forgive other people when they sin against you, your heavenly Father will also forgive you. But if you do not forgive others their sins, your Father will not forgive your sins." (Matthew 6:14–15, NIV)

My mother taught me the power of forgiveness before she passed. My mother came to faith after a childhood marked by alcoholism, poverty, and abandonment by her father. In writing her obituary weeks before her passing, my mother scolded me because I left out her father's name.

"But he abandoned you," I replied in my defense. "He was never the father he should have been."

"But he was my father," she said. "I've forgiven him."

My mother taught me in that moment that forgiveness goes a long way—all the way to the cross. She was able to forgive the father who abandoned her and caused her so much pain because *God* had forgiven *her*. She had made the decision to extinguish the bitter flames that singed her heart.

Dr. David Jeremiah instructs us to reject bitterness for harm that's been done to us and instead fight for joy at any cost, knowing that God will serve justice.[9] Unforgiveness only hurts the one who harbors it. It's like a poison that travels through the body and occupies the heart, and the only antidote is to let it go and forgive. Trust that *God* will make all things right in *His* time.

As undeserving recipients of the greatest forgiveness—the one God offered through the sacrifice of His Son—we also must extend forgiveness to those who have hurt us. We must also go to those whom we've hurt and ask *their* forgiveness. Then the healing begins.

Why Should I Worry?

Why worry? "Because it gives me something to do" is not a good answer. Worry wreaks havoc on our bodies while getting us nowhere. It's like a rocking chair in motion—it goes back and forth but makes no forward progress. That's why the Bible instructs us to cast our cares on Him and instead pray about all our concerns:

Be anxious for nothing, but in everything by prayer and supplication, with thanksgiving, let your requests be made known to God. (Philippians 4:6)

After my oncologist warned me I would lose every hair on my body, I prepared myself for physical changes. I'd never had short hair except as a child. It was suggested that I adapt to a shorter look in stages. But my hairdresser gently said, "It's less devastating if you come back after the first chemo and allow me to shear your head."

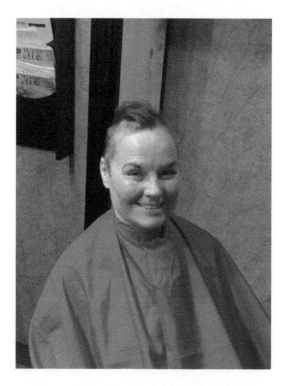

I decided to try a Mohawk first!

The Bible says that a woman's hair is her glory (1 Corinthians 11:15). My glory was soon scattered all over the floor. Frankly, my looks were the least of my worries. I shifted into survival mode and focused instead on my brain, heart, and lungs. Hair loss was just a small inconvenience. I simply picked out a wig, a few hats, and some scarves to cover my head.

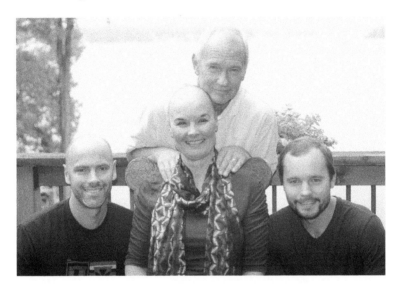

With Joshua, Alton, and Harrison Brant. The baldest one wins!

Jesus tells us not to worry but to live one day at a time (Matthew 6:25–34). Cancer forced me to do just that.

Let's look at a breakdown of the things we tend to worry about:

- 40 percent of the things we worry about never happen
- 30 percent we can't do anything about
- 12 percent are worries about health (which can cause health problems)
- 10 percent are petty, miscellaneous concerns
- 8 percent are real, legitimate problems[10]

Such a small percentage of our worries are legitimate concerns. We must learn to pray about our concerns, make adjustments for the things we cannot change, and let the rest go. My counseling advice for worrying clients was always, "If there is something you can do about it, do it. If not, pray about it."

Do not worry but, rather, have faith in God and who He is. Worry is a sign that you doubt God's sovereign will in your life. Laura Harris Smith says, "Doubts are splinters in the fingers of your faith; they prevent you from taking a firm grip."[11]

When we keep our eyes focused on Him, we are able to walk through the trial or fire without being consumed because His presence is with us.

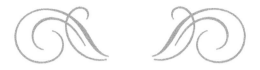

CHAPTER 9

God's Remedies for Healing Emotions

Your problems are temporary, but God's promises are eternal. His promises will outlive your problems and carry you to heaven, where there are no problems, no pain, no death, no tears.
—David Jeremiah

Your physical health is influenced by your thought life. When you spend your time thinking negative thoughts and giving place to negative emotions such as fear, doubt, anger, resentment, and unforgiveness, it will have a negative impact on your health and well-being.

The opposite is also true. When you think positive thoughts and give place to uplifting emotions such as laughter, hope, and joy, these will impact your health in a positive way. The word *enthusiasm* comes from a Greek word meaning "God within." Even on the cancer journey, you and I can be shining lights of God's power within us.

The Bible encourages us to maintain a positive attitude. For example, the apostle Paul instructs us in Philippians 4:8 to dwell on, or think about, good things—things that are true or noble or pure or lovely. Proverbs 23:7 directly hints at the power of our thoughts: "For as [a person] thinks in his heart, so is he." Today, medical research has repeatedly shown the positive and negative effects that emotions have on the human body.

Of all people, God's children have good reason to be positive *whatever* our circumstances. Nevertheless, God has graciously given all of us powerful ways to manage our feelings and relieve the stresses that can destroy our health.

The Awesome Power of Prayer

Many cynics believe that prayer is a waste of time, but the Bible speaks of prayer as an important discipline in our lives. It's part of our daily communion with God, a conversation between two people who love each other. Prayer is where we pour out our hearts, confess our sins, make our needs known, and listen as He speaks to our hearts.

According to the Gospel Coalition, there are 650 prayers in the Bible and 450 recorded answers. The New Testament records Jesus praying twenty-five times during His earthly ministry.[1] In 1 Thessalonians 5:17, we are told to "pray without ceasing," and in Philippians 4:6 to "be anxious for nothing, but in everything by prayer" make our requests known to God.

The movie *War Room* depicted prayer as a powerful weapon in life's battles. My own life has taught me the value of daily, consistent prayer. Sometimes we can't see or feel God working, but my experiences have shown me that He's working on our behalf even before we utter a prayer— going before us, just as He promised, providentially putting into motion events and supplies to meet our needs in the coming days.

When I was just a teenager, I repeatedly prayed for my father and family without knowing if God heard. Twenty years later, I cried tears of joy as I realized God had been working behind the scenes to bring my father to his knees and my family to faith and healing as I prayed. My father eventually dedicated his life to the Lord and left his legal and political career to enter full-time lay ministry with my mother. God then led him to post-communist Romania, where he helped the underground church plant on the surface and the government to come to freedom. Only God could make this possible!

Prayer also calms the mind and the emotions, which is important because an emotional and stressed brain causes an excess of cortisol to be produced in our bodies. Too much cortisol results in elevated inflammation in the body and fat around the belly while literally wearing out the immune system.[2]

When first diagnosed, I remained quiet about my cancer journey. Only a few people were aware of my condition. But before my first surgery, I felt the need for prayer support. That night, I sent an e-mail to close friends and family informing them of our situation and asking for prayer. This prayer support would prove to be an important part of my success along the way.

Laughter Is the Best Medicine

During a vitamin C infusion after my first surgery, my brother Jack came to see me. He was in Chicago on business and had come a day early to check on his ailing sister. Jack and I both possess a keen sense of humor. As we were leaving the infusion bay, I caught a glimpse of my hair after surgery.

"Oh my, my hair is a mess," I said.

Jack pulled out his comb. "Try this," he said.

As I tugged the comb through my tangled mess, a rumble began in my little toe and spread to my entire body. I looked at Jack and said, "Here I am, in the middle of a . . . cancer . . . center . . . where most people don't have any . . . hair . . . and I'm worried about my hair!"

That's all it took for both of us to lose control. We were both close to falling on the floor in uncontrollable laughter. I could barely walk, but I was holding my gut as if it might burst.

Laughter is good for the soul, and we often find it in the strangest places in the middle of a crisis. Maybe it seems strange to you that cancer patients would find anything funny about their situation, but laughter is part of the journey. Not only is it an emotional release, but laughter is in fact a powerful medicine that actually increases blood flow and oxygenation, reduces stress, and boosts the immune system! A study conducted at Loma Linda Medical University found that just one hour of watching a humorous video increases the activity of a person's natural killer cells, B cells, T cells, and immunoglobulins, with the effects lasting up to twelve hours![3]

According to a fifteen-year study on the link between sense of humor and mortality involving more than 50,000 women and men, Norwegian researchers suggested that laughter actually helps a person to live longer! The findings showed that women with a strong sense of humor have a 48 percent lower risk of death from all causes, including a 73 percent lower risk of death from heart disease. Mirthful men have a 74 percent lower risk of death from infection.[4]

Charlie Chaplin, perhaps the greatest of all comics, is widely quoted as saying, "Laughter is the tonic, the relief, the surcease for pain." Indeed, laughter causes your brain to release a flood of endorphins, which supercharge the immune system and can possibly slow down cancer. According to Mike Adams, author of *The Five Habits of Health Transformation*, "When you laugh, you generate a wealth of healing biochemicals. For every minute of laughter, you produce somewhere around $10,000 worth of healthy body chemistry."[5]

According to the Cancer Treatment Centers of America, laughter therapy may provide benefits such as:

- Enhancing oxygen intake
- Stimulating the heart and lungs
- Relaxing muscles throughout the body
- Triggering the release of endorphins
- Easing digestion and soothing stomachaches
- Relieving pain
- Balancing blood pressure
- Improving mental functions
- Reducing stress and tension
- Promoting relaxation and sleep
- Enhancing the quality of life and sense of well-being[6]

With a ha-ha-ha, a ho-ho-ho, and a couple of tra-la-las, Dorothy and her friends laughed the day away at the end of a long and arduous journey. And humor helped my husband and me to survive my cancer journey. I believe our Lord has a sense of humor, and He expects us to have one, too. "He will yet fill your mouth with laughter and your lips with shouts of joy" (Job 8:21, NIV).

The Healing Benefits of Music

Before my first surgery, a nurse reminded me that I would need to be awake for this procedure. The radiologist began meticulously placing wires through my right breast to mark where both tumors were. This would serve as a guide for my surgeon, helping her not to waste any precious tissue.

The nurse gave me earphones and offered to play music to calm my fears. "What kind of music do you prefer?" she asked.

"Contemporary Christian," I replied.

The first song that played was "I Am Not Alone" by Kari Jobe. The song speaks of how God is always with us as we walk through trials in life. Before I knew it, peace and comfort were circulating throughout my body. I breathed a sigh of relief. The words and sounds helped me to endure this sensitive and invasive procedure.

At age 70, Joni Eareckson Tada is one of the oldest living quadriplegics in the world. Her love for music and its ability to lift her spirits is one of the secrets to her longevity. I don't know anyone who's faced tough times with such grace. Music has served her as a healing agent for many years through multiple trials, including cancer. Joni's favorite songs are hymns that minister the words of God to her soul.

A study by Tenovus Cancer Care and the Royal College of Music found that singing in a choir for just one hour reduces stress, improves mood, and boosts levels of immune proteins in people affected by cancer.[7] According to the National Center for Biotechnology Information (NCBI), music therapy has the potential to improve neurodegenerative and neuropsychiatric disorders by creating new brain cells and neural connectivity.[8] Music can also restore hormonal and immunological balance.[9]

Well-chosen music has the power to console us in our depression and liberate us from despair. As with Joni, music has ministered to my soul during dark and challenging times. "Tell Your Heart to Beat Again" by Danny Gokey is another song that carried me through my cancer journey.

Stress Reduction App

There are many ways to reduce stress, including exercising, walking, singing or listening to music, taking a long bath, gardening, writing, crafts, playing with a pet. You must find the activities that work best for you.

Dr. Tim Wiles, a health coach who gave advice at my school, recommended the HeartRate+ app to all teachers dealing with stress. This app is designed to help balance your sympathetic and parasympathetic nervous system to protect your body from the impact of stress. When CTCA's Mind and Body Clinic recommended the same app to reduce my stress levels, I downloaded it to my phone. It's now a regimen I practice once or twice daily depending on my current stress load.

You simply open the app and place your index finger over the camera of your phone. While breathing deeply in time with the moving ball on the screen, you are developing coherence between your heart rate and your breathing. I try to get my coherence in the 60–80 range. It takes only five minutes per session.

I look back on the fifteen years of grief while caring for parents as they passed on. I wish I had added this regimen to my walking and singing. For the amount of stress I was experiencing, I did not do enough to protect my health.

Standing on Hope in Our Trials

Hope is a great motivator; despondency is a great killer. When in the middle of a crisis, it's easy to forget that the current trial may one day be something we look back on and thank God for. Hope was one of the essential traits I taught children as an elementary school counselor. The Core Essentials Curriculum defines hope as "believing that something good can come out of something bad." That's Romans 8:28 in a nutshell.

My father, Harry Dent, and the late Chuck Colson both looked back on a nation's scandal called Watergate—a dark and scary time in their lives—and thanked God for it. Anything that causes you to find salvation and leads you to your God-given purpose in life is a blessing. I can now say that cancer was the best thing that ever happened to me.

In the midst of my cancer journey, the notion that my disease was a blessing was the furthest thing from my mind as I rode the roller coaster ride of emotions. When I began to see the light at the end of the tunnel, I started to recognize the many things I'd learned about my faith, my body, and what's truly important in life. That's a blessing!

When you're walking through the valley of the shadow of death, you need only to look up to the other side to know that you'll be back on top. And if your cancer journey proves to be your "ticket to heaven," then celebrate and bless your loved ones before you move your permanent address to an eternal destination. And if you have no assurance of salvation, there's never a better time to read your Bible and seek God.

Dr. Viktor Frankl, a Holocaust survivor and author of *Man's Search for Meaning*, pointed to having hope and a mission to fulfill as reasons some prisoners survived the great atrocity. Hope is a powerful motivator. We must never forget that most trials are temporary.

Living Life with an Eternal Perspective

Life is so much more than the here and now. Since my cancer diagnosis, I have come to fully appreciate and understand that none of us is promised tomorrow. But we *are* promised something far more important—eternal life—*if* we're willing to take hold of it (John 11:25).

When I interviewed Joni Eareckson Tada, she told me that when she received her first cancer diagnosis, she wondered if this might be her ticket to heaven. As I've mentioned, my elderly mother felt the same way when she was diagnosed. She put up a good fight, but when there was no longer hope for recovery, she had her bags packed and her thumb out. She was ready for that sweet chariot to sweep down, pick her up, and carry her home.

The guarantee of heaven and eternal life with Christ is another reason we, as Christians, should remain joyful and positive even in the midst of life's toughest trials. This brings to mind my friend Jane Hartwell's mother. As she was dying from cancer, she blessed each of her children and grandchildren before she entered the Pearly Gates. This is the attitude we should all have—trusting that God will care for the loved ones we leave behind.

Keeping our focus on eternity takes the sting out of fear. It enables us to look at life both from God's perspective and through the lens of eternity. Those trials that burden us and steal our joy become a mere dot on the infinite line of eternity. My pastor likes to say, "We are to live for the line, not the dot."

We must reassess every trial we encounter in the light of eternity. Looking at it this way, my cancer diagnosis becomes my opportunity to see God work in my life. It could set the stage for a miracle, helping others, or it could be *my* ticket to heaven! If you have a prodigal child, it could be that the road they're on is what God will use to bring them back to Him.

It's no wonder God's Word instructs us to be joyful in hope, patient in times of trouble, and always faithful in prayer (Romans 12:12). We need to build our lives around things that are eternal—the Word of God, people's souls—and live each day in light of eternity.

The Power of Love

It's no secret that happily married couples live longer, and that people who have close social interactions and emotional support tend to be healthier. Love and support are critical for the patient in the cancer journey.

I scheduled my first MRI for a day when my husband could be with me. In my later years, I've developed claustrophobia. When I laid prostrate on that MRI bed with arms extended and the technician slowly backed me into the dark tunnel, my skin moistened, and my heart danced to an uncomfortable beat. The imaging device started hammering away with what sounded like machine gun fire, and my happy-go-lucky attitude vanished. "Get me out now!" I screamed.

The technician had other patients waiting. "If you can't do this now, we'll need to reschedule you weeks later, when your doctor can order you a sedative," she explained.

So, I went back in to avoid delay, but lying face down in that tunnel for fifty minutes was unbearable. I felt as though I was being buried alive.

"I need my husband," I said.

"We don't usually allow this," the technician said, "but if you think it will help, I'll get him."

I've never been so relieved to see Alton's face. I reluctantly laid down, and she backed me into the abyss once more. Alton grabbed my right hand and lovingly caressed it throughout the ordeal. His protective touch calmed the turmoil within and helped me make it through the storm.

If cancer patients have a spouse, significant other, or friends and family who unconditionally love and support them during the cancer journey, their chances of survival increase. I was blessed to have all three. On the Yellow Brick Road, my husband was my Tin Man, the man of steel with a heart as big as the world. He lifted me up when I needed it and loved me even when I was at my worst. As a result, my journey has given me a heart for others like me.

The opposite is also frightfully true. Think of those cancer patients who are abandoned by a spouse because of their illness. These individuals need their friends, family, and church to rally around them because feeling loved and accepted helps the body heal.

Consider oxytocin, a powerful hormone that acts as a neurotransmitter in the brain. It's often called "the love hormone." One of the natural ways of increasing the body's oxytocin production is through human touch. This hormone triggers the bonding between a mother and an infant at birth, for example, and plays an active role in developing trust, creating empathy, handling stress, and controlling depression and anxiety. Positive hormones like oxytocin and serotonin are your allies in the cancer journey.

We always need the affection of other people, but friends and loved ones are particularly important when we're feeling down for the count. Remember when the flying monkeys attacked Dorothy's friends and left the Scarecrow in pieces strewn about the Haunted Forest? The Lion and the Tin Man wasted no time in reassembling their friend. Scarecrow was able to get back on his feet and continue the journey for one reason: A community of true and trusted friends and loved ones put him back together again in his time of need.

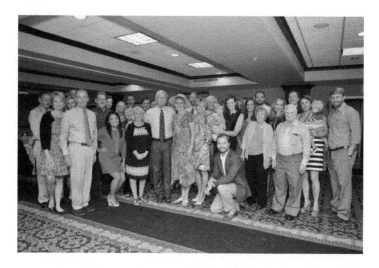

Friends and family throw us a surprise 40th anniversary party after my 5th chemo.

My Recommendations for All

Due to the far-reaching impact of emotions and faith on our physical health, my list of recommendations is the same for everyone, whether or not you're currently experiencing the cancer journey. If you want to be healthy, you must learn to manage your emotions, build your faith, and actively participate in a loving community of friends and family.

My recommendations are:

1. Take the ACE test and allow the Word of God and godly counsel to penetrate those adverse experiences in your life.[10]
2. Allow God's strength to work through your weaknesses.
3. Confess your sins daily to the Lord. Be realistic about your part in your physical and spiritual health and commit to making lifestyle changes.
4. Do not harbor resentment and unforgiveness; it can only hurt you. Practice a life of forgiveness.
5. Live one day at a time, pray about your worries, adjust to the things you can't change, and continually lay your concerns at the foot of God's throne.
6. Wield prayer as a powerful weapon in the battles of your life.

7. Before reacting in anger, try deep breathing, exercise, self-control, and godly expression of your feelings.
8. Play music to calm your mind and body and minister to your soul.
9. Cultivate the gift of laughter to lighten your load.
10. Use the HeartRate+ app to reduce stress.
11. Stand on the hope and promise that God will use your trials and difficulties for His glory and your good.
12. Look at your current troubles from an eternal perspective.

For those who have faith in Christ, cancer is just a dot on the line of eternity. We are meant to live for the line, not the moments and maladies that dot our relatively brief lives on earth. There is a place over the rainbow where cancer and problems will exist no more. It's called heaven, the final destination for those who love the Lord. There we will be given glorious new bodies that will never wear out. It's the land we all long for and dream of—an eternal home. Yes, Dorothy, there is such a place.

STEP SIX:

THANKFULNESS

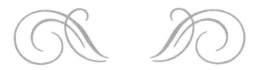

CHAPTER 10

Practicing Gratitude as an Attitude

Be anxious for nothing, but in everything by prayer and supplication, with thanksgiving, let your requests be made known to God; and the peace of God, which surpasses all understanding, will guard your hearts and minds through Christ Jesus.
—Philippians 4:6–7

A wise man should consider that health is the greatest of human blessings, and learn how by his own thought to derive benefit from his illnesses.
—Hippocrates

My job as a school counselor was to give students the support and skills they needed to be successful in school and in life. I planned my guidance lessons around character development, which was lacking in many homes. One of the character traits that was high on my list was gratitude.

I taught kids the value of gratitude using the story of the Pilgrims and the hardships they endured in the New World. They experienced fear, sickness, starvation, unimaginable loss, grief, and grueling work during the coldest of winters. Yet they gave thanks to God after the most devastating year of their lives.

At our home, Thanksgiving is much more than just spending time with family while sharing food. Thanksgiving is the time when we individually express to one another what we are thankful for. Although the holiday comes once a year, expressing gratitude regularly is a brain-healthy practice that can change your brain and bring you joy year-round.

Chick-fil-A's Core Essentials Curriculum is a character education program they've developed for use in schools. This program defines *gratitude* as "Letting others know you see how they've helped you." The curriculum includes a teaching song called "Gratitude Is an Attitude." I thought of this song often during my father's journey and passing from Alzheimer's disease, my mother's journey and passing from cancer, my husband's journey with prostate cancer, and of course my own cancer journey.

We should be in the habit of expressing gratitude to others for what they bring to our lives, but we need to make a daily priority of counting our blessings and "giving thanks *always* for *all things* to God the Father in the name of our Lord Jesus Christ" (Ephesians 5:20, emphasis mine). A grateful heart is a healthy heart. Here are just a few of the many Bible passages on the importance of keeping an attitude of gratitude:

> Devote yourselves to prayer, being watchful and thankful. (Colossians 4:2, NIV)

> Enter into His gates with thanksgiving, and into His courts with praise. Be thankful to Him, and bless His name. For the Lord is good; His mercy is everlasting, and His truth endures to all generations. (Psalm 100:4–5)

> For although they knew God, they neither glorified him as God nor gave thanks to him, but their thinking became futile and their foolish hearts were darkened. (Romans 1:21, NIV)

Writing a Gratitude List

What's good for the pupil is good for the teacher. During thirty-two years of counseling students and parents through various crises in their lives, my advice always included writing a gratitude list. My cancer journey provided the opportunity for me to swallow a bit of my own medicine.

So, after the toughest year of my life, here was my gratitude list:

- God will use this for good
- My husband, family, and prayer network who supported me
- The doctors and staff who lovingly cared for me at CTCA
- I survived five surgeries with no complications
- I survived the harshest of chemotherapies with minimal side effects
- After chemotherapy, all bloodwork returned to normal ranges within six weeks
- God's provisions for our expenses
- I lived to see my son get married and have his first child
- I'm still alive and well on planet Earth!

My biggest blessing during the journey was the encouragement and support of my husband. It was difficult to look at myself in the mirror after the surgeries and chemo robbed me of my femininity. But Alton's love never waned. "You're the prettiest gal east of the Mississippi," he'd say. The Tin Man is awarded his heart for demonstrating true love—putting the needs of others ahead of his own. That's why I call Alton my Tin Man.

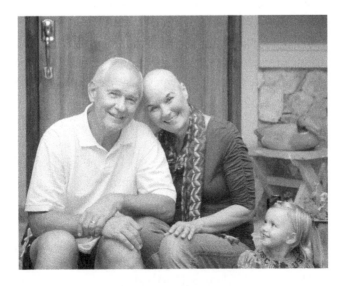

Sullivan Brant witnesses her grandparents' gratitude for each other.

I will always be thankful for all the staff at CTCA, who helped me beat cancer. In some of my lowest moments, the nurses, aides, and drivers held my hand, prayed with me, and offered me a word of cheer. I've never experienced an entire hospital so focused on patient care. And my progress is proof. How many chemo patients have you seen hiking mountains or snow skiing after receiving chemotherapy treatments?

Why Gratitude Is Important

Using images from SPECT scans of the brain, Dr. Daniel Amen found that practicing gratitude causes real physiological changes that enhance brain function. He says, "People who practice gratitude are healthier, more optimistic, make progress towards their goals, have a greater sense of well-being, and are helpful to others."[1]

His study showed that negative thoughts can deactivate specific regions of the brain associated with motor coordination, thus causing a person to be clumsier. His scans also indicated that important structures like the cerebellum, the frontal lobe, and the temporal lobes were deactivated when people focused on what they hated about life. He concluded, "Where you bring your attention, determines how you feel and how your brain performs. Your thoughts can make you feel great or make you feel sad, forgetful, and clumsy." Practicing gratitude activated these same structures and calmed the emotional brain.[2]

Amen is one of many doctors who are promoting the daily expression of gratitude as a lifestyle practice. He suggests that gratitude is better than Prozac because it has an upside but no downside.

A 2015 *Newsweek* article cited research showing grateful people tend to be more hopeful and healthier, enjoy improved sleep quality, have increased self-esteem and empathy, and show higher levels of resilience.[3]

According to the research of Dr. Robert Emmons, "Gratitude increases happiness and reduces depression." In fact, gratitude blocks many toxic emotions that destroy happiness.[4]

Dr. P. Murali Doraiswamy, head of the division of biologic psychology at Duke University Medical Center, proclaims, "If thankfulness were a drug, it would be the world's best-selling product with a health maintenance indication for every major organ system."[5] According to Dr. Doraiswamy, studies have shown how the expression of gratitude leads to measurable beneficial effects on multiple body and brain systems. These include mood neurotransmitters (serotonin, norepinephrine), reproductive hormones (testosterone), social-bonding hormones (oxytocin), cognitive and pleasure-related neurotransmitters (dopamine), inflammatory and immune systems (cytokines), stress hormones (cortisol), cardiac and EEG rhythms, blood pressure, and blood sugar.[6]

Psychologist Renee Jain recommends a well-known and researched exercise to get out of a negative rut and improve psychological, social, and physical health—the Three Blessings Exercise. You simply write down three good things that have happened to you that day. "Studies reveal," Jain says, "that those who continue this exercise for one week straight can increase their happiness and decrease depressive symptoms for up to a six-month period."[7]

The Doctor Prescribes:

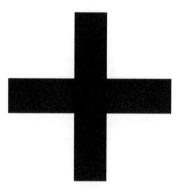

Being Thankful

I believe that if you truly have faith in your heart, gratitude must naturally follow. One cannot be positive or thankful enough. Gratitude helps to promote healing in the body by activating mood neurotransmitters, lowering blood pressure, decreasing cortisol in the body, and improving blood glucose levels. A thankful, content person is a healthier person.

Dr. Robert L. Elliott

Controlling Envy with Blessings

Jealousy and envy can eat us alive. William Shakespeare called jealousy "the green-eyed monster."[8] Envy is the sin of not loving our neighbors because they have something we want and do not have, and it's among the deadliest of sins. In fact, the very first murder was the result of envy (Genesis 4). What does this have to do with cancer, you ask? Proverbs 14:30 (NIV) says, "A heart at peace gives life to the body, but envy rots the bones."

James identified envy, jealousy, and covetousness as the source of so much of the war and conflict we experience within ourselves and with others (James 4:1–2). The apostle Paul gave us the key to beating these sins:

> I have learned to be content whatever the circumstances. I know what it is to be in need, and I know what it is to have plenty. I have learned the secret of being content in any and every situation, whether well fed or hungry, whether living in plenty or in want. I can do all this through him who gives me strength. (Philippians 4:11–13, NIV)

There will always be someone who has more than you, just as there will always be someone who has less than you. Most of the poor in America would be considered wealthy in many parts of this world. The key to defeating jealousy and envy is to turn your covetousness into thanksgiving and praise God for what you *do* have. If you have basic food, clothing, and shelter, consider yourself blessed. If you are free of pain and relatively healthy, consider yourself blessed. If you are able to work, consider yourself blessed. When you concentrate on your many blessings, you don't have time to be envious of others.

The Path to Peace

The Bible commands us in Ephesians 5:20 to give thanks "always for all things." Bestselling author Ann Voskamp believes that counting your blessings is a way of reorganizing your brain to focus on goodness. At times, when the path in life is dark and difficult to follow, the only way through is to focus on the light—the good things.

In a talk in which she extolled the physical benefits of practicing a lifestyle of gratitude, Voskamp noted:

> On the night Jesus was betrayed, He broke bread and gave thanks. If Jesus can give thanks in that, we can give thanks in anything. If Jesus chooses gratitude to destroy evil, do you have a better weapon? Gratitude amplifies goodness so you can hear the grace of God. Gratitude amplifies the light of God so you can see the face of God in the midst of the dark.[9]

Trees need harsh winds to challenge them, as this causes their roots to grow deeper into the soil, which in turn will support the tree as it grows taller. Likewise, adversity helps a person to grow strong; our roots won't grow deep if everything always goes our way. Turning to God in times of adversity helps us to draw closer to our Father as we gain something of His perspective and learn to trust His sovereign will in our lives.

Of course, we have a choice of where we turn our attention. As Christians, we are to look for "good things" and dwell on these (Philippians 4:8). And we are to be thankful for the good we find. After all, "every good gift and every perfect gift is from above," from "the Father of lights" (James 1:17). Certainly, we of all people have the most to be thankful for, given the promise of eternal life to come.

In Philippians 4:6–7, Paul makes an interesting connection between thankfulness and peace of mind:

> Be anxious for nothing, but in everything by prayer and supplication, *with thanksgiving*, let your requests be made known to God; and *the peace of God*, which surpasses all understanding, will guard your hearts and minds through Christ Jesus. (emphasis mine)

Whatever our circumstances, when we make our requests known to God with a heart of thanksgiving, we can have peace of mind to a quality and extent that "surpasses all understanding." Peace of mind, like other positive emotions, promotes healing in the body, as though the cells in the body are eavesdropping on our prayers and drawing strength from the supernatural peace we receive from God.

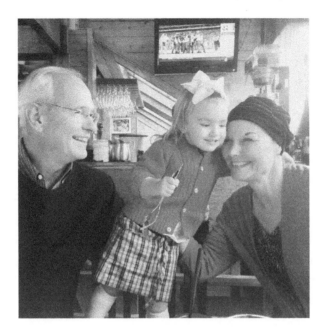

After seeing her Gigi and her many looks during cancer, Sullivan
Brant says, "You're my Gigi with the crazy hair!"

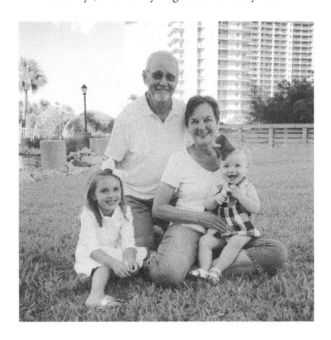

What a blessing to live to enjoy both Sullivan and Ashlen Brant!

My Recommendations

Because gratitude is an attitude and costs us nothing, my recommendations are the same for all:

1. Every day, give thanks and praise to God, even if you're in the middle of the cancer journey. Recognize that gratitude and a cheerful heart are good medicine.
2. Always express your thanks to those who help you.
3. Make a gratitude list daily. Count your blessings and look for the silver lining behind every cloud.
4. Don't allow envy and jealousy to control your life. Learn to be content whatever your circumstances.
5. Pray continually, making your requests known to God with thanksgiving.

King Solomon wrote, "A cheerful heart is good medicine, but a crushed spirit dries up the bones" (Proverbs 17:22, NIV). One of the most enduring heroines in literature and film, Dorothy Gale, remained cheerful undeterred by her circumstances. Despite being lost and far from home, threatened by powerful forces she didn't understand, she kept a cheerful disposition that drew others to her as if she were a magnet. Dorothy made lifelong friends within moments of meeting them in part because she made a habit of always looking for the good things along her journey. And so should we. The apostle Paul instructs us to dwell on "the good."

STEP SEVEN:

DETOXIFICATION

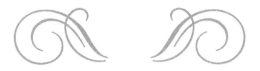

CHAPTER 11

Reducing Environmental Toxins

Then God blessed them, and God said to them, "Be
fruitful and multiply; fill the earth and subdue it; have
dominion over the fish of the sea, over the birds of the
air, and over every living thing that moves on the earth."
—Genesis 1:28

Then God saw everything that He had
made, and indeed it was very good.
—Genesis 1:31

Ninety-five percent of cancer is caused by
a poor diet and excessive toxins.
—Columbia University School of Public Health

From the beginning, God gave mankind the responsibility to "subdue" the earth and have "dominion" over it (Genesis 1:28). He also put man in the Garden of Eden "to tend and keep it" (Genesis 2:15). Many have differed over exactly what these passages mean, but it seems clear that God has instructed us to be responsible in caring for His creation.

Francis Schaeffer wrote, "The Christian is called upon to exercise dominion without being destructive."[1] John Calvin interpreted "dominion" to mean that we are to care for and keep the earth in a manner that does not neglect, injure, corrupt, mar, or ruin the earth.[2] The late Billy Graham said, "The Bible clearly commands us to protect our environment in Genesis 2:15. It is wrong for us to misuse our environment."[3]

While conducting research after my cancer diagnosis, it became abundantly clear to me that we are not properly caring for the earthly home God has given us. We must do better. Certainly, we suffer very real consequences when our water is unclean, our air is too polluted to breathe, and our food is poisoned with toxic chemicals.

Time to Clean House

God created a perfect environment in the Garden of Eden. Fast-forward to present day and the earth is significantly different. We've not been proactive in protecting the planet, and we're all paying the price.

Author and naturopathic physician Dr. Joe Pizzorno defines a toxin as "anything that interferes with human physiology." He believes the primary cause of chronic disease today is environmental toxins. Toxins are contributing to the rise in diabetes and can alter how our genes are expressed. Pizzorno says that the synergistic adverse effect of multiple toxins together is particularly powerful.[4]

According to Dr. Don Colbert, "Lead has actually contaminated our entire planet. Lead has even been found in some of the most remote areas on the planet such as the Arctic Ice Cap and in the New Guinea aborigines that live far away from any sources of lead exposure."[5] I was personally stunned when high levels of lead were found in my body through testing done several years before my cancer diagnosis.

Dr. Mark Hyman, director of the Cleveland Clinic Center for Functional Medicine Institute, recently said, "Our toxic load is greater than any time in human history with over 80,000 chemicals developed since the 1900s."[6]

In fact, the Environmental Protection Agency's Toxic Release Inventory of 2012 reveals that 3.63 billion pounds of toxic chemicals were released into our air, water, land, and disposal sites in 2012.[7] We now have over 3,000 chemicals in our food supply, with new chemicals being produced each year. Pesticides used in farming have been linked to lower sperm counts in men[8] and higher amounts of xenoestrogens in women. Colbert says, "These counterfeit estrogens are more potent than the estrogen made by the ovaries, and they can have a stimulating effect on breast and other hormone-related cancers."[9]

The U.S. Centers for Disease Control (CDC) has reported there are approximately 140 toxic chemicals now present in our bodies. Even more alarming, these toxins are implicated in 70 percent of all chronic diseases![10] In a study spearheaded by the Environmental Working Group (EWG), researchers found an average of 200 industrial chemicals and pollutants in umbilical cord blood from ten babies born in U.S. hospitals in August and September of 2004.[11]

Thankfully, God created our bodies with filtering systems built into the skin, liver, colon, kidneys, and lungs. But just like a car with a dirty air filter, our filters get overloaded. However, there are things we can do to lighten the load, allowing our filtering systems to perform their God-intended functions.

Ty Bollinger, who began researching causes and treatments of cancer after he lost his parents and relatives to the disease, started *The Truth About Cancer* movement. Although his movement is controversial to some, I've learned much from his research. Bollinger claims, "The root cause of nearly all disease—cancer, diabetes, heart disease—is an overload of toxins and chemicals accumulating inside your body. Period."[12]

Toxins are all around us. They're in the foods we eat, the water we drink, the air we breathe, the cleaning agents we use, and the cosmetics and lotions we put on our skin. Many of the chemicals in these products did not exist until the middle of the twentieth century, so our bodies are constantly being exposed to many toxins that our great-grandparents didn't face. Given the serious rise in cancer rates in recent years, we must reduce our *toxic load*. Toxic load is the accumulation of poisons that burden the body's organs, thus causing our built-in filtering systems to overload.

Toxins in Our Food

The demand for organic foods has increased dramatically in the past decade. In fact, Costco is now planting its own organic fields and adding more organic products to its offerings. Amazon has acquired the leader in the market, Whole Foods, and is now shipping organic foods to your door. According to the Organic Trade Association, organic sales in the U.S. totaled nearly $50 billion in 2017, and demand continues to grow.[13]

True confession: I never ate organic until I was diagnosed with cancer. I assumed my body could filter out whatever minimal chemicals I consumed. What I didn't realize was that an accumulation of chemicals was overloading my system.

Perhaps you've seen the video case study about the Palmbergs, the Swedish family of five who ate conventional food for one week and organic for two weeks while providing urine samples to researchers. The results were dramatic. The lab found a number of insecticides, fungicides, and plant growth regulators in the Palmbergs' samples during the first week. After shifting their diet to organic foods, researchers found little evidence of pesticides and other compounds in their urine samples.[14]

According to Dr. Joshua Axe, organic foods contain more vitamins, minerals, enzymes, and micronutrients than conventionally grown foods. By eating organic, you avoid dozens of chemical pesticides and herbicides linked to various health problems, environmental destruction, and antibiotic resistance.[15]

There are currently 3,000 high-risk toxins, including pesticides, which by law are excluded from use in growing certified-organic products. Eighty percent of the antibiotics sold in America are used to raise livestock and poultry. Axe believes that this is fueling the appearance of antibiotic-resistant germs that are difficult to kill. Meat products certified organic by the USDA come from animals that have been fed zero antibiotics or growth hormones. Animals are also fed organically, while having access to the outdoors and being raised according to strict animal health and welfare standards.

Foods labeled organic are also guaranteed not to be genetically modified. Many genetically modified foods contain high amounts of pesticides. In fact, many are genetically modified specifically to withstand being sprayed multiple times with chemicals. Every weed around that plant may die, but when you eat the food from that plant, you are biting into a scrumptious load of toxic chemicals. Food for thought.

The Mayo Clinic has also taken note of the benefits of choosing organic foods, citing increases in nutrients and flavonoids, higher omega-3 fatty acids in dairy and meat, lower cadmium levels in grains, and lower detectable levels of pesticide residue.[16]

A cancer friend who had months left to live because her chemo was not working, asked her oncologist, "What would you do if you were me?" His reply was telling: "I'd try eating organic. The research is showing it may help." Good advice but sadly a little late.

The BreastCancer.org website is now bringing this information to light. Their report "Nine Steps to Eating a More Healthy Diet" says, "To reduce your exposure to pesticides, you might want to buy organically grown food and organically produced dairy products."[17]

Hormones regularly show up in our dairy products, chicken, beef, plastic bottles, and the lining of cans containing Bisphenol A (BPA), which mimics the hormone estrogen. If a cow is given hormones, she will produce more milk and meat. The same goes for chickens and their production of eggs. But this approach is short-sighted, as these hormones are passed on to those who consume these products. We simply aren't using common sense at a time when estrogen-fed cancers continue to rise.

Yes, it costs more to eat a diet of organic foods, but I now believe it's worth the extra it saves in health benefits. My cancer treatment cost $600,000; eating organic would've cost far less.

The Environmental Working Group (EWG) website provides a helpful guide to choosing fruits and vegetables according to their expected chemical content. The EWG analyzes pesticide studies and ranks forty-five of the most popular fruits and vegetables according to their average pesticide content. According to the EWG's 2019 Shopper's Guide to Pesticides in Produce, the following are the "Dirty Dozen," the twelve most contaminated fruits and vegetables. These are the products that typically contain the highest amount of chemicals, with strawberries being the most contaminated:

The Dirty Dozen

1. Strawberries
2. Spinach
3. Kale
4. Nectarines

5. Apples
6. Grapes
7. Peaches
8. Cherries
9. Pears
10. Tomatoes
11. Celery
12. Potatoes

Does this mean you should avoid all strawberries, apples, and spinach? Absolutely not! But these are food products you should definitely seek out from organic or local trusted growers only.

The EWG's "Clean Fifteen" is a list of fruits and vegetables that can be eaten sensibly without worrying about chemicals and pesticides, especially when you are eating out. NOTE: These lists are updated from time to time on the EWG website; check there for the most current information. Here is their 2019 Clean Fifteen:

The Clean Fifteen

1. Avocados
2. Sweet corn (some are GMO)
3. Pineapples
4. Frozen sweet peas
5. Onions
6. Papayas (some are GMO)
7. Eggplants
8. Asparagus
9. Kiwis
10. Cabbages
11. Cauliflower
12. Cantaloupes
13. Broccoli
14. Mushrooms
15. Honeydew melons[18]

Dr. Don Colbert advises that fruits and vegetables with thick peels and skins usually contain fewer pesticides.

Toxins in Our Water

Earlier we discussed the many health benefits of proper hydration. Following the water crisis in Flint, Michigan, where high levels of lead were found, you must ask yourself, *Is my water source clean enough?* An investigation by *The Washington Post* has led many to believe the problem is more widespread than we think.[19]

Ocean Robbins of The Food Revolution Network claims, "By not taking the time to research our water, countless people are placing themselves and their families at risk for a variety of devastating side effects, including cancer." According to Robbins, lead is not the only contaminant we should be concerned about. Chromium-6, the cancer-causing chemical made famous in the movie *Erin Brockovich,* is contaminating water supplies of more than 75 percent of all Americans.[20]

Most chemicals that are sprayed on our foods and lawns, dumped in our landfills, or emitted into the air eventually end up in our water. Why? Rains wash these chemicals into our lakes and rivers, allowing them to seep into our groundwater. Other dangerous pollutants showing up in our drinking water include drug residues from antibiotics, antidepressants, hormones from birth-control pills, and painkillers.

The presence of so many dangerous chemicals in our tap water is why so many people are turning to bottled water. Sadly, it has proven to be no safer.[21] Dr. Axe reports, "In widespread testing, a whopping 93 percent of bottled water samples tested were contaminated with tiny pieces of plastic." It's no wonder Axe calls bottled water "toxic rip-offs."[22] Bottled water is often full of endocrine-disrupting chemicals,[23] and it comes with increased cancer risk according to a recent study showing that eleven out of eighteen bottled waters sampled induced estrogenic effects in a human cancer cell line.[24] A 2009 study revealed that the estrogen contamination in bottled water originated from compounds leaching from the packaging material. Warm temperatures accelerate this effect.[25]

But that's not all. Testing conducted by the EWG found popular bottled water brands containing mixtures of thirty-eight different pollutants, including bacteria, fertilizer, Tylenol, industrial chemicals, kerosene, styrene, mold, yeast, and algae.[26]

So, if our tap water is unsafe and bottled water is no better, where do we turn for the crucial hydration of our bodies? The twofold answer lies in 1) filtering your own water at home and 2) using glass, steel, and ceramic containers to store and drink water.

Fluoride may help fight tooth decay, but do we need to bathe in it and drink it all day? Fluoride can suppress thyroid function, and thyroid disorders are more prevalent where water is fluoridated. Chlorine prevents bacteria from growing in our water supply, but it too can damage your ability to process thyroid hormones. The thyroid, the body's master regulator, controls many functions vital to prevent cancer. Consider it your responsibility to filter out these chemicals and pollutants at your kitchen sink. Your water company does the best they can and delivers water that is safe from bacteria, but they can't guarantee you 100 percent pure water.

Spring water from a pure source is the best water for your body, but it can be expensive. Many experts recommend drinking water that has been filtered using reverse osmosis. Other people use a Berkey Water Filter, which sits on your counter and is priced at less than $350.

After my cancer diagnosis, Alton and I installed a whole-house water filter in our home and a reverse-osmosis filter beneath our kitchen sink. By stopping the flow of many chemicals into our bodies via our water supply, we've greatly reduced our toxic load.

Toxins in the Air

According to Dr. Joseph Pizzorno, "Over 6.5 billion pounds of chemicals are released into the air every year."[27] There are toxins in the air. There are estrogens in the air. The closer you live to the inner city, the more pollutants there will be in the air you breathe.

Air pollutants come from many sources such as chemical sprays, manufacturing byproducts, automobile emissions, smoke and debris from wildfires, and fertilizer fumes. Nevertheless, it's common sense to research the area where you live and the air quality there and make some tough decisions for the sake of your family's health.

One of the checks we did in our home after my cancer diagnosis was a radon test. Radon is a naturally occurring radioactive gas that can cause lung cancer. Our home had slightly elevated levels of the gas—enough that we chose to install a radon-removal system. Radon is more prevalent in areas where the underlying bedrock is granite.

Indoor Toxins

Studies by the Environmental Protection Agency (EPA) reveal that indoor air pollutants can be two to five times higher than outdoor levels.[28] Because the most toxic exposure you experience may be in your own home, consider opening your windows whenever possible. Indoor air pollution is caused by a combination of particles such as dust, pollen, pet dander, mold spores, and smoke. These are combined with ozone, invisible gases, and volatile organic compounds emitted by building materials, furniture, carpeting, paint, and cleaning and personal care products.

The Consumer Wellness Center just released a list of 700+ chemical formulas found in Tide laundry pods. Many of these chemicals are considered extremely toxic to human health.[29] I strongly suggest that you examine your cleaning products and remove any that increase the toxic burden on your body.

Because weather sometimes makes opening the windows of your home prohibitive, you might want to invest in some highly rated air filters or a whole-house or room filtering system. My two favorite room filters are Austin Air and Air Doctor Purifier, because these can filter both common types of indoor pollution. I can't always control what's in the air I breathe, but I have taken decisive steps to filter the air in my own home.

I also needed to reduce the chemicals in my home. I now either make my own cleaning supplies, or I purchase plant-based products sold in stores. Method, Meyers, Seventh Generation, and doTERRA make many cleaning products (for reasonable prices) without toxic chemicals.

I threw out the normal bathroom cleaner (just read the ingredients on the label). I no longer clean my Jacuzzi tub with bleach; I simply use vinegar and baking soda. I've also ditched my lawn weed killer. I simply pull those weeds or spray them with an all-natural solution.

Toxins in My Mouth?

When I first heard medical doctors and dentists talk about the toxicity of mercury amalgam fillings, I began telling my dentist to only use porcelain or white ceramic in my crowns and fillings. As a child, my addiction to sugar left me with a mouthful of cavities.

Twelve years ago, I needed a root canal. I thought nothing more about it until I began hearing numerous testimonies from both patients and doctors about the procedure's possible long-term dangers. Few doctors would argue with the notion that oral health is foundational for systemic, or whole body, health. Now there is mounting evidence that root canals can endanger the body by laying the groundwork for future disease both inside and outside the mouth.

Then again, why should I be worried if I have no symptoms? That was my philosophy until I heard the personal testimony of a man whose health had greatly deteriorated but was restored after a holistic dentist removed his root canals. His situation caused me to dig deeper.

When it was time for my breast thermogram, I asked the technician to take a few pictures of my jaw in the area where I had had a root canal performed. I was shocked when the image showed a line of inflammation running from the bottom of that root canal, cascading down toward my right breast!

I immediately called Dr. Gary McCown in Knoxville, Tennessee, and scheduled a consult exam. Dr. McCown is an award-winning dentist, researcher, and adjunct professor at the University of Tennessee College of Dentistry. During the consult, I showed him my thermogram results.

"I'm not surprised," he said. "I see this frequently. And let me guess, was your cancer in this right breast?"

"Yes," I replied, "but I had no symptoms. The x-ray showed nothing."

"Root canals are not the best way to treat a tooth in this condition," he said. "The tooth must be pulled and replaced by an implant or bridge. Root canals and subsequent possible cavitations can contribute to and be a cause of systemic disease."

A deeper dive into this common dental procedure reveals that root canals can foster harmful bacteria by creating an oxygen-free environment perfect for anaerobic bacteria to thrive after dentists seal off the treated area. These bacteria-harboring toxins can leak into surrounding tissue and pick up a free ride to any location in the body.[30]

"It must be removed," Dr. McCown told me. I agreed, and he proceeded to remove my root canal. When he removed the cap from the crown of the tooth, a pungent smell permeated the room. "Is that coming from me or you?" I mumbled, trying not to gag.

"That's the smell of accumulated bacteria," he replied. "Those toxins have kept your lymphatic system on your upper right side working overtime."

Most breast cancers start on the left side, but mine had started on the side where my lymphatic system (part of the immune system) was under constant attack. After the area healed from the removal of the root canal, another thermogram showed that the line of inflammation was gone.

I had learned the painful lesson that dental health impacts the body in often unseen ways. I only wish I'd discovered this sooner and had been more proactive in caring for my teeth.

Toxins from Cosmetics and Personal Care Products

The most eye-opening scientific fact I've learned from both my husband's and my cancer journeys is that whatever touches the skin is absorbed into the bloodstream and circulates throughout the body. In fact, it's estimated that 60-70 percent of the chemicals we apply to our skin are absorbed into our bodies. Before cancer, I always assumed that as long as I washed those chemicals off at some point, I was fine. Think again!

I also didn't carefully read the labels on my skin care products and cosmetics. The average woman in the U.S. uses about twelve personal care products, while the average man uses about six. Many of these products contain petroleum, phthalates, lead, aluminum, DBP, DEA, PPD, triclosan, parabens, and various carcinogens.

Phthalates are especially common in health and beauty products, except in Europe where they are banned. In fact, the European Union has banned almost 1,000 chemicals that are allowed in the U.S. in personal care products. Companies in the U.S. are not even required to list all their product ingredients.

Phthalates are known endocrine disruptors. They interact with the endocrine receptor sites located on every cell in your body and can mimic or stimulate estrogen production in the body. Phthalates are found in nail polish, perfumes, and plastic wrap. Parabens, which serve as preservatives in many cosmetics, are also endocrine disruptors. Both should be avoided.

When I learned there might be hazardous chemicals in my makeup and personal care products, I went to the EWG website to search their Skin Deep database. I realized that the makeup and skincare products I had been using for more than twenty-five years contained many dangerous ingredients. Ironically, the woman who started this cosmetic company died from breast cancer.

I have now switched entirely to cosmetics that contain no phthalates, parabens, lead, or other chemicals. I favor companies such as Juice Beauty whose products are made from natural ingredients. Coconut oil and jojoba oils are now my favorite moisturizers for face and body.

Toxic Exposure in One Day

If you're still not convinced that most of us are bearing a high toxic load, consider for a moment an average American woman's daily schedule. After waking:

- We take a shower or bath with soaps and shampoos containing sodium lauryl sulfate and propylene glycol in water that contains fluoride, chlorine, and a number of other chemicals.
- We dry off with a towel that has been washed in 1,4-dioxane, quaternium-15, and diethanolamine.
- We apply skin lotion that contains methylparaben, propylparaben, and polyethylene glycol.
- We use deodorant containing aluminum chlorohydrate and isopropyl alcohol.
- We apply mousse containing alcohol, glycerin dimethyl ether, benzophenone-4, and copolymer to add volume to our hair.
- We use hairspray with alcohol and octinoxate isophthalates.
- We apply face creams and anti-aging creams containing hydroquinone and BHA.

- We sculpt our face with a foundation containing polymethyl methacrylate and finishing powder containing talc.
- We spray our bodies with cologne or scented perfumes that contain acetone, benzyl acetate, ethanol, and methylene chloride.
- We eat a hearty breakfast of dairy products containing antibiotics and BHT hormones and wheat products containing high amounts of gluten and pesticides. We drink coffee that contains pesticides and herbicides. We often use plates and cups made from plastic and Styrofoam, allowing more chemicals into our bodies, especially if we use a microwave.
- After breakfast, we brush our teeth with toothpaste containing triclosan, sodium lauryl sulfate, and fluoride (which is not good for those with thyroid problems). We then rinse with mouthwash containing alcohol, methylparaben, and chlorhexidine.
- We get dressed in clothes that have been washed in chemicals and treated with wrinkle-resistant chemicals such as formaldehyde, fire retardants, and dry cleaning chemicals such as perchloroethylene. When we perspire because we're running late, these chemicals can leach into our skin.
- We start the car and drive to work while breathing the gasoline fumes from other vehicles.
- Throughout the day, we meet our daily hydration goals by drinking water containing chlorine, fluoride, and other chemicals.
- We wash our hands before lunch using an antibacterial soap containing triclosan or benzalkonium chloride.
- For lunch, we eat a hamburger and fries containing chemicals, hormones, additives, and preservatives. Our soft drink contains many chemicals and loads of sugar and contributes to our body's acidity.
- After lunch, we reapply our lipstick that is tainted with lead and polymethyl methacrylate.
- We light a scented candle with paraffin wax to dispel the odors in our office, but it gives off benzene and toluene.
- On the drive home we fill up our car with gas, breathing fumes while standing at the pump. Occasionally, we spill gas on our shoes and bring the fumes into the car.

- Now and then we stop at the salon to get our hair colored using treatments loaded with chemicals such as synthetic hair dyes from petroleum or coal tar sources, formaldehyde, diethanolamine, and monoethanolamine. Any chemical that touches our head is circulated through our blood to all parts of the body.

- While waiting for the coloring chemicals to set, we get our nails done with treatments that include huge amounts of toxic chemicals such as phthalates, formaldehyde, and toluene. Nail polish removers generally contain acetone, so just sitting in a nail salon is hazardous to our health.

- When we arrive home from work, we notice ants in the kitchen. So, we grab the insecticide and spray the room with chemicals such as cypermethrin and imiprothrin.

- We microwave a farm-raised salmon dinner loaded with chemicals on a plastic dish. Or we may sauté that salmon in our Teflon-coated or aluminum cookware which also releases chemicals into the food.

- Once a week we clean the bathroom while inhaling toxic chemicals such as DEG mono-n-butyl ether, benzene, and chloroform.

- When it's time for bed, we might put on a nightie that has been treated with flame-retardant chemicals and fabric softener containing alpha-Terpineol and ethanol. We then apply a soothing ointment to our nose and lips—an ointment that contains petroleum.

I hope this little checklist helps you to visualize the number of toxins our bodies are exposed to daily. Yes, we all carry a toxic load whether we can see it or not. And when our toxic bucket is full, our immune system suffers.

Even the American Cancer Society, who for years had been denying the link between toxins and cancer, now says, "Compounds in the environment that have estrogen-like properties are of special interest. For example, substances found in some plastics, certain cosmetics and personal care products, pesticides, and PCBs (polychlorinated biphenyls) seem to have such properties. In theory, these could affect breast cancer risk."[31]

However, you can reduce your toxic burden by eating organic as much as possible, drinking filtered water, using plant-based products in your personal care and cleaning products, and using traps instead of insecticides to get rid of bugs and pests. Some things are more difficult to control, such as the building products where you work and the air you breathe, but you can be mindful of fumes when pumping gas by starting the pump and walking away until the tank is full.

Here is a before-and-after list of products I used before my cancer and the switch I made thereafter:

Toxic Product Before Cancer	Less Toxic Substitution After Cancer
Toothpaste	Tom's, doTERRA, or DIY (do it yourself)
Cosmetics	Juice Beauty, Beautycounter, or plant-based
Anti-aging products	doTERRA or DIY (I make my own using essential oils)
Ointments	Badger Winter Wonder Balm and Coconut Oil
Household cleaning products	Meyers, Seventh doTERRA On Guard, and DIY
Comet	Bon Ami
Candles for odors	Essential oil sprays
Deodorant	Mineral stones, Tom's, Native, DIY creams
Pest sprays	Peppermint oil in water sprayed; also pest traps
Teflon or aluminum cookware	Stainless steel, glass, and ceramic cookware
Plastic bottles and storage	Glass bottles and steel storage containers
Tide Laundry Pods	doTERRA, Seventh Generation, Method, or DIY
Dishwasher and dish soap	Seventh Generation, Method, Meyers, or DIY
Soap and shampoos	Organic or DIY
Hairspray and gels	John Masters (organic), Aveda (less toxic)

There are many websites such as Dr.Axe.com, Dr. Eric Z, and The Prairie Homestead.com that provide do-it-yourself recipes for personal care and home cleaning supplies that use natural ingredients. I now make my own shampoo, laundry detergent, dishwashing soap, and skincare creams. I only make those items that don't require cooking. For skin care, I use jojoba and coconut oils as my base and add oils such as myrrh, frankincense, lavender, and rose.

When bees invaded our home, I did a little research and added a few drops of peppermint oil to water in a spray bottle and used that instead of poison. I knew I'd achieved victory when my neighbor called to say he saw hundreds of bees leaving my home! Oils such as rosemary, thyme, basil, melaleuca, and peppermint can also be used in spray bottles in your garden to ward off pests.

Many grocery stores now carry organic food, and the number is growing yearly. My best source is the Ingles that is closest to my home. Publix, Aldi, Kroger, Safeway, and others also carry many organic dairy, fruits, vegetables, and meat products. Costco has the best price for organic ground beef, chicken, frozen fruits, nuts, and produce.

Yes, my grocery bill has gone up. But I encourage you to look at your food as medicine and a way of reducing your toxic burden. By doing this, your healthcare bills should be lower. Compared to surgery and chemotherapy, the cost of eating organic and avoiding chemicals is a drop in the bucket.

Reducing your toxic load is a preventive action that can save you thousands in the future. If you don't spend time and money on your wellness, your time and money will be spent on your illnesses. Concentrate on reducing your chemical intake realizing that up to 90 percent of toxins may be coming in through our mouths through food and water[32] as opposed to achieving perfection. There's no such thing as perfection in this imperfect world. But we must do what we can to protect ourselves from the environment around us.

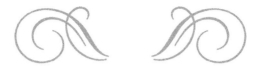

CHAPTER 12

Detoxing to Reduce Your Toxic Load

Again He said to me "Prophesy to these bones, and
say to them, 'O dry bones, hear the word of the Lord!
Thus says the Lord God to these bones: "Surely I will
cause breath to enter into you, and you shall live.
I will put sinews on you and bring flesh upon you,
cover you with skin and put breath in you; and you
shall live. Then you shall know that I am the Lord."'"
—Ezekiel 37:4–6

After my chemotherapy regimen was ended, I returned to see Dr. Passini to check on my lead levels. Even before my cancer diagnosis, my body had shown high levels of lead, a known carcinogen. Five years ago, my levels were at 40; under 4 is considered normal. By the time of my cancer diagnosis, I had lowered my lead levels to 19.

After the recheck, I knew the news wasn't good when Dr. Passini summoned me to her office. My lead levels were unchanged, but I was not prepared for the news that followed. Dr. Passini cautiously slid my results across her desk. "Your mercury levels are now very high, as are your platinum, gadolinium, aluminum, and uranium levels."

As I glanced over the results, tears began to flow. There was a new battle before me due to the many poisons that had been used to kill the cancer cells. I would now have to remove the toxic metals and chemicals from my body before they created other cancers and diseases. I was only halfway to the Emerald City.

Dr. Passini attempted to encourage me by outlining a plan of metal detoxification over the next few years. She also suggested I look into using an infrared sauna to complement the IV chelation treatments that would pull the metals from my body.

On the long drive home, I kept pulling off the road to cry. The battle was not over, but I was too weary to fight. My usual spunk had been buried in a toxic dump, while the Cancer Witch was writing in the sky, "Surrender!"

Never. I may go down for a spell, but not for long. I am a fighter, and I was not about to let this news get the best of me.

I began researching heavy metals and detoxing. I examined every type of infrared sauna to find the best one. I volunteered to take part in a clinical trial measuring the levels of toxic chemicals in my body before and after repeated sauna use.

After eating organic for a year and changing out my personal care products and cosmetics to safer choices, my initial test results showed four of twenty areas in the red, or high, zone. I focused my efforts on using my sauna to reduce these four areas.

I had high levels of 2,4-Dichlorophenoxyacetic acid (2,4-D), a common herbicide that was a part of Agent Orange, the notorious defoliant chemical used by the U.S. in the Vietnam War. It's commonly used to grow genetically modified foods and as a weed killer for lawns. This herbicide is also a known endocrine disruptor, and it can block hormone distribution and cause glandular breakdown. A later test revealed I had high levels of glyphosate, another pesticide used on GMO crops. This was fascinating to me since I had been diagnosed with an estrogen-fed breast cancer.

My toxic chemical profile also revealed ultra-high levels of MTBE and ETBE, which are gasoline additives acquired through inhalation or skin exposure to gasoline and exhaust fumes. We quickly removed the gas cans, lawnmower, and gas-powered tools that were stored in the garage under our bedroom. I also changed how I pump gasoline by turning my head upstream from the fumes and walking away while the gas is pumping.

My body also contained high levels of perchlorate (PERC)—found in bleach, fertilizers, and rocket fuel—and diphenyl phosphate (DPP), which is found in flame retardants.

On the other hand, my test results were encouraging in that sixteen of the twenty areas tested were in the green, or low, zone. My new goal was to reduce all toxic metals and chemicals in my body to safe levels. With the help of my Clearlight Infrared Sauna, and a detox specialist, my levels are now all in the low range, allowing my immune system to work as God intended. Praise God!

The first step in detoxification is to reasonably avoid your exposure to harmful chemicals. The second step involves removing the toxic load you have accumulated over time. Let's look at some effective ways to achieve this.

The Doctor Prescribes:

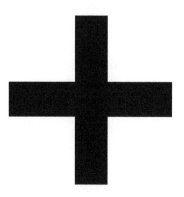

Reducing Your Toxic Load

Hydration and good renal function will help reduce your toxic load. Environmental toxins may in fact play a damaging role, but most people cause their own personal toxic load through poor dietary habits and a sedentary lifestyle. You also need to beware of toxicity caused by antibiotics, which are commonly used during cancer therapy. Not only has the overprescribing of antibiotics resulted in resistant strains of harmful bacteria—antibiotic resistance is one of the most urgent threats to public health—but antibiotics can also damage normal mitochondria and destroy a person's gut microbiome. The condition of your mitochondria is key to your health, so exercise caution and don't pressure your doctor to give you an antibiotic next time you have a cough.

Dr. Robert L. Elliott

Dry Brushing and Natural Fibers

After chemotherapy, the nurse who performed my thermogram recommended I start dry brushing my body. Dry brushing is an inexpensive process that involves moving a dry brush over your body in slow, circular motions two to three times a week. The firm bristles of the brush exfoliate your skin while stimulating your lymphatic system to do its most important job—cleaning cells and dumping toxins into the blood, so they can be eliminated.

Simply buy a body brush and begin brushing with light strokes on the bottom of your feet. Always brush towards the heart and continue until you've covered all the skin. Sensitive breast tissue can be manually massaged. This only takes five minutes.

Wearing clothing made from natural fibers is also a good idea because natural fibers allow the skin to breathe and detox. I now look for organic cotton as much as possible, especially when shopping for garments I wear next to my skin or sleep in at night. Other natural fibers include wool, flax, hemp, and silk. I also found some reasonably priced organic cotton sheets on the Target website.

Reducing Toxic Load through Exercise and Sweat

Exercise is another inexpensive way to stimulate the lymphatic system to take out the body's trash. Exercise also aids the body in removing toxins via sweat. In fact, anything that causes you to sweat—exercise, steam room, sauna, etc.—helps to remove toxins that have accumulated in your body.

The day my infrared sauna arrived, I ripped it out of the box. It was like receiving an early Christmas gift. Hundreds of doctors recommended infrared sauna as one of the best ways to sweat out heavy metals and toxins from your body. After eighteen months of using my sauna three times a week on average, my platinum and gadolinium levels have reduced by over 75 percent. My uranium, lead, and aluminum levels have fallen by 25 to 40 percent each.

I highly recommend the use of an infrared sauna. My husband also uses it one to two times per week as a form of prevention. The sauna, hydration, and exercise are key ways to reduce toxins in the body through your largest detox organ—the skin.

Please check, however, with your health practitioner before using the infrared sauna. Cancer patients who have had multiple lymph nodes removed are not usually advised to use a sauna. You must also check with your doctor before using a sauna if you have any serious disease such as uncontrolled high blood pressure, heart failure, cardiac arrhythmia, chronic lung disease, or poorly controlled diabetes.

Here is my detox protocol with the sauna:

1. Drink several glasses of water before, during, and after sauna.
2. Do 30 minutes of moderate- to high-intensity exercise.
3. Dry brush the body.
4. Detox in the sauna for 30–40 minutes. (Start at 15 minutes and build up from there.)
5. Shower with cool water to close pores, so toxins are not reabsorbed into the skin.
6. Hydrate with a dash of Himalayan or Celtic salt in water to replenish trace minerals lost while sweating.

Using Coffee to Detox

Dr. Max Gerson used natural treatments such as organic juices to activate the body's extraordinary ability to heal itself. Gerson is famous for his coffee enema protocol, and many holistic practitioners recommend this protocol today. After cleansing the large intestine with warm water, coffee is inserted into the body through the rectum. The coffee stimulates the liver to produce glutathione, which cleanses the bile ducts where many toxins are stored.

Don't laugh. Enemas are one of the oldest medical treatments, dating back to Egypt in 1500 BC. Coffee enemas appeared in the medical literature as early as 1917 and remained in the *Merck Manual of Diagnosis and Therapy* until 1972. German scientists discovered that coffee was able to open the bile ducts and increase production of bile, which then stimulated the liver to detox the body and excrete the toxins through the digestive tract.

Daily and Bi-Yearly Detox

With the marked increase of toxins and chemicals in our environment, many health practitioners are recommending both daily and periodic detox regimens. My daily detox involves proper hydration, exercise, lots of clean fruits and vegetables, and an early morning detox drink. Here's the drink that starts my day on the right detox pathway:

Daily Detox Drink

1–2 Tbsp. of Bragg's Apple Cider Vinegar
1–2 tsp. of raw honey
1–2 Tbsp. of freshly squeezed lemon
Dash or two of red cayenne pepper
8 ounces of warm water
Stevia packet, if needed
You can add one drop of lemon essential oil and On Guard Oil Blend by doTERRA to build your immune system.

Every six months, Alton and I go all out with a thirty-day cleanse where we eat all organic foods while avoiding sugar, meat, dairy, gluten, etc. completely. Our regimen allows for a smoothie or two each day using high-powered greens and cleansing fruits. Since the foods are in the form of smoothies, this allows our bodies to put their energy toward cleansing and healing instead of digestion.

Vitamin C Infusions to Reduce Toxic Load

Oxidative stress is created when there are more toxins and free radicals present than the body has defenses to neutralize them. For example, if you have inflammation, you have increased oxidative stress and vice versa. Oxidative stress is thought to be involved in the development of many diseases including ADHD, Parkinson's, Alzheimer's, heart disease, chronic fatigue, and cancer.

Enter vitamin C. It's the muscle of the immune system—the main fuel by which immune cells do their jobs. Dr. Thomas Levy reports, "Vitamin C works to either encounter the toxin before it does its oxidative damage and neutralize it, or it donates electrons to restore the cell to normal biological function."[1]

Dr. Paul Marik made national headlines when he successfully used vitamin C intravenously with B[1] and cortisone in a last-ditch effort to cure a patient dying of sepsis. According to Dr. Ron Hunninghake of the Riordan Clinic, more than 900 doctors in Japan are using vitamin C infusions. Now Harvard, Beth Israel, and Johns Hopkins are studying C's effects on sepsis.[2]

The University of Iowa,[3] Cornell,[4] and Jefferson University[5] are researching the benefits of and using IV vitamin C as an adjuvant with chemotherapy. In this way, they are able to reduce the dosage of chemotherapy and achieve better outcomes with fewer side effects.[6] Vitamin C infusions given before and after chemotherapy made a profound difference in my own cancer journey.

Benefits of Intermittent Fasting

Intermittent fasting is when one abstains from eating and drinks only water for twelve to sixteen hours. This means if you finish dinner at 6 p.m., you don't eat again until between 6 and 10 a.m. the next morning. According to Dr. David Jockers, the powerful benefits of intermittent fasting include:

- Boosting weight loss
- Promoting the secretion of the Human Growth Hormone (HGH), which reduces triglycerides, boosts HDL, and stabilizes blood sugar
- Improving genetic repair mechanisms
- Improving immune regulation
- Stimulating autophagy[7]

Autophagy (literally "self-eating") is a natural regeneration process in which the body rids itself of old, damaged cells and recycles them for energy.

Autophagy also restricts viral infections and cancer cell development while protecting cells from toxicity and chronic inflammation.

Deep Breathing, Herbs and Essential Oils

I began deep breathing as a form of therapy from the moment I was diagnosed with cancer. Deep breathing helps to detoxify the body. At night, I diffuse an essential oil blend of eucalyptus, melaleuca, peppermint, and others to help open up and heal my lungs.

I also began drinking smoothies made of organic fruits and vegetables to help my lungs heal and to speed up the detoxification of my body after I was declared cancer free. My lungs are improving, and I no longer need an inhaler.

Here is my smoothie recipe. Substitute one cup of blueberries for the grapes if cancer is still present in your body:

Recipe for Grape Pomegranate Peppermint Smoothie for 2

    2 cups organic grapes
    4–6 ounces pomegranate seeds (fresh or frozen)
    2–3 drops oil of peppermint
    1–2 Tbsp. ground flax seeds
    1 scoop Organixx or Ancient Nutrition vanilla bone broth protein powder
    1 Tbsp. coconut oil or several avocado chunks
    Handful of broccoli or other sprouts
    1–2 cups of spinach, kale, or other greens
    2 cups coconut water, almond milk, coconut milk, or filtered water
    ½ cup of coconut or milk yogurt
    Fresh mint leaves
    ½ cup ice (optional)[8]

Prevention on a Budget

As stewards of the earth, we have not been proactive in protecting the home that God gave us. Our world and our daily lives are full of toxic chemicals, and we're all paying the price. My recommendations for detoxifying your life and your body are:

1. Filter your drinking water. Also, stop drinking from plastic bottles and containers. Use glass, ceramic, or steel containers instead.
2. Use the EWG's Dirty Dozen list as a guideline for replacing the most toxic fruits and vegetables with organic alternatives and gradually increase your intake of organic foods.
3. Buy organic dairy and meats as your budget allows. Find a local farmer or food co-op as a source. Buy a freezer to buy cheaper in bulk. Try growing some of your own food and herbs without the use of toxic pesticides.
4. Examine and change out any personal care products containing toxic chemicals. To save money wait until a product is empty and then swap it out for a smarter choice.
5. Phase out the use of plastics in food storage and aluminum foil and aluminum cookware in baking. Use glass, ceramic, and stainless steel instead.
6. Consider the proximity of your hair products to your brain and gradually change over to organic options for shampoo, gels, and coloring.
7. Make some of your own personal care and cleaning products to save money and lessen your toxic load. Refer to my list of alternatives and find your own substitutions.
8. Consider intermittent fasting to prevent and treat illnesses, including cancer.
9. Start the day with my detox drink to keep your liver clean and fully functioning.

Remember that your goal is to reduce—not remove all—toxins so your immune system has fewer distractions.

In the Cancer Journey

In addition to the above recommendations, you must do of all *these* immediately:

1. Install a whole-house water filter and reverse osmosis at your kitchen sink to stop toxic exposure when bathing and drinking.
2. Eat mainly organic foods—including fruits, vegetables, meats, and dairy, as well as wild-caught seafood. If you are receiving chemotherapy, don't add any more chemicals to your toxic load!
3. Limit anything that touches your skin—including cleaning products, makeup, and skincare—to nontoxic substances, realizing that around two-thirds of what goes on your skin enters your bloodstream. Again, avoid adding any more chemicals during chemotherapy.
4. Keep your bowels moving through the use of enemas, exercise, hydration, MiraLAX, etc.
5. Use dry brushing, exercise, and other activities that promote sweating and stimulate the lymphatic system. Check with your doctor as to when it is permissible to dry brush when taking chemotherapy.
6. Use deep breathing, smoothies, herbs, and essential oils to detoxify your body.
7. Consider a daily and bi-yearly detox protocol to reduce the toxins that accumulate in your body.

Going All Out

If you have the financial resources, I recommend taking these additional steps:

1. Consider buying an infrared sauna to use in your home two to three times a week after treatments are over or join a gym that has one.
2. Consider buying a whole-house air filter or at least a filtering machine for your bedroom, where you spend a third of your day.

3. Wear natural fibers whenever as possible. Buy sheets, pillowcases, sleepwear, and undergarments made of 100 percent cotton.
4. Find a doctor who administers vitamin C infusions (cost: $200 each).

I made an oath to myself, "If I ever get my body cleaned out, I'll never pollute it again." This approach is critical to living a long, healthy life. My body was a living scrapyard of accumulated metals and chemicals. Don't give the Wicked Witch the upper hand. Diminish her power by taking away her broom—that is, her ability to distract your immune system. Detoxing helped me to restore my body after chemotherapy. It gave breath to my dry bones.

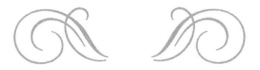

CHAPTER 13

The Invisible Toxin

Put on the whole armor of God, that you may be able to stand against the wiles of the devil.
—Ephesians 6:11

A wise man is strong, yes, a man of knowledge increases strength.
—Proverbs 24:5

Human-made electromagnetic fields (EMFs) are a relatively new health concern. Since electricity and electric lights were first introduced into homes, our exposure to EMFs has dramatically increased. Twentieth-century appliances such as refrigerators, toasters, microwaves, vacuum cleaners, washers, dryers, cordless phones, and televisions all create EMFs. In recent years, families and businesses have come to depend on widespread new technologies such as cellular phones, computers, and Wi-Fi, all of which involve the generation and proliferation of energy fields.

What does this have to do with your health? First of all, electrical currents are part of the human body's functioning. For example, an entire network of nerves is always relaying signals to the brain and back again in the form of electrical impulses. Also, nearly all the body's billions of cells generate electricity through the movement and rearrangement of charged particles, and these electrical currents allow the heart muscle to contract at the right time. Any disruption in these electrical activities can lead to illness.[1]

Given the ubiquitous presence of mobile phones and Wi-Fi signals in our culture, many healthcare professionals are now becoming concerned about the impact of electromagnetic radiation and how it affects our bodies. Many believe that when human-made energy fields react with the electrical impulses in the human body, the body can become confused and trigger a fight-or-flight response. When the body is constantly in fight-or-flight mode, the result is exhaustion, which can weaken or compromise the immune system. When I interviewed Alfred Hanser, co-founder of GIA Wellness, he compared the body's constant bombardment by EMFs to a boxer in a prizefight. He said, "It's one thing to get hit occasionally, but when you are repeatedly hit night and day, it's hard for your body to recover."

It's something I never considered until my cancer journey. My husband and I had wondered about the impact of Wi-Fi signals and cell phone EMFs, but it's not something you can see, taste, or smell like cigarette smoke. For years, we simply ignored it, but no more. I now call EMFs "the invisible toxin," because their invisibility causes us to dismiss them as harmless when they're not.

We can't live today without these technologies, but we must use common sense to protect our immune systems from being constantly pummeled like an overmatched boxer in the ring. There's no way we can move off the grid, unless you want to live in a Faraday cage. Maybe twenty years ago it was possible, but not today. However, we must realize that radiation—even in the form of cell phones and Wi-Fi—will gradually wreak havoc with our immune systems.

Alfred Hanser of GIA Wellness explained to me that scientists used to think that as long as radiation was not heating and met certain IEEE standards, we would be safe. But today we are beginning to connect years of cell phone use to brain tumors, breast cancer, and reproductive issues. I remember what political strategist Lee Atwater told my dad before Atwater died of a massive brain tumor. "Harry," he said. "I can't help but believe there's a connection between the fact that my brain tumor is right below the place I constantly put my cell phone." And no one used his cell phone 24/7 as did Lee Atwater.

Dr. Veronica DeSaulniers of BreastCancerConqueror.com made a believer out of me when she showed a slide of a thermogram taken of a man's head after a fifteen-minute cell phone conversation. The entire side of his head was inflamed! I also saw a picture of a young child where an MRI showed major inflammation from cell phone use, which expanded much further in her head due to softer tissue. It's widely known that chronic inflammation over time can cause DNA damage and lead to cancer.

If you don't believe me, get out your cell phone and go to "Settings," then "General," then "About," and scroll down to "Legal," then "RF Exposure." Your cell phone manufacturer recommends using a hands-free option to reduce your exposure to RF energy.

What EMF Research Is Telling Us

No one is more adamant about the dangers of cell phone radiation than Dr. Devra Davis, an epidemiologist and Founding Director of the Center for Environmental Oncology. Davis has more than 200 publications to her name and currently lectures at Harvard. She was one of the first scientists to recognize the dangers of secondhand smoke and recommended that smoking not be allowed in public places.

When first approached about the dangers of EMFs, Davis dismissed the question as ridiculous. But as she explored the matter, she began to see similarities in stages to her research about secondhand smoke and admitted she was wrong. She now lectures worldwide on EMFs and warns that with six billion cell phones in use today, these issues must be addressed.[2] Canada and Belgium are among the countries now developing regulations to address these concerns. In 2011, the alarm was sounded when the International Agency for Research on Cancer (IARC) declared cell phones a Class B carcinogen.[3]

Davis believes we must learn more about the physical effects caused by this form of radiation. Her greatest concern is EMFs' impact on young children. The younger the child, the more radiation is absorbed because their skulls are softer than those of adults and their brains contain more fluid. Davis also believes that cell phone radiation produces free radicals that weaken DNA, the blood-brain barrier, and cell membranes.

A study done by the Cleveland Clinic in 2008 indicated that men who carry cell phones tend to have lower sperm counts: "Results suggest that the use of cell phones by men is associated with a decrease in semen quality. The decrease in sperm count, motility, viability, and normal morphology is related to the duration of exposure to cell phones. More studies are needed to identify the mechanism involved in the reduction of semen quality."[4]

Ladies, warn your husbands. But considering a woman's breast is mostly fat and body fluid, and cell phones are a two-way microwave radiation that penetrates fats and fluids easily, we must also be cautious. There are now reports of women who repeatedly stored their cell phones in their bras for many years developing tumors right below that position.

Dr. Lisa Bailey, a breast cancer surgeon and former president of the California division of the American Cancer Society, warns, "We have seen some very unusual breast cancers in both young women with no risk factors, and postmenopausal women who have carried their cell phones close to or in their bras. So a microwave signal close to the body might have an effect on your breast tissue."[5] Dr. Bailey also directs us to the fine print that comes with your cell phone:

> Carry iPhone at least 10 mm away from your body to ensure exposure levels remain at or below the tested levels.[6]

This lesson was made all too clear to me when a friend of mine from high school was diagnosed with breast cancer. She had a known habit of putting her cell in her bra for years. Her doctor declared this as the likely cause of her cancer.

Dr. Andrew Goldsworthy of the Imperial College in London believes that the hormone glands are particularly sensitive to radiation. He said, "Although electromagnetic fields frequently stimulate glandular activity in the short term, long-term exposure is often harmful in that the gland ceases to work properly."[7]

Dr. Davis's recommendations include:

- Avoid carrying any mobile phone on your body.
- Avoid holding any mobile phone against your body when in use. Use speakerphone or an "air tube" earpiece.

- Avoid using your cell phone when the signal is weak, because additional radiation is emitted for the signal to reach a tower.
- Put your mobile phone on "airplane mode" when it's not in use or on your body.
- Avoid using a mobile phone in cars, trains, planes, or elevators as these magnify the radiation all around you.
- Keep mobile phones away from you when sleeping and charging.[8]

Technology to the Rescue

Dr. Igor Smirnov's successful breakthrough with MRET-Activated Water (see chapter 2) inspired him to develop another MRET invention. This invention superimposes electromagnetic noise fields onto a radiation wave to counteract the biological effects of harmful electromagnetic radiation. The patent for an Electromagnetic Shielding Material Device was issued to Dr. Igor Smirnov in 2007.

Some companies are now manufacturing cell phone cases designed to block radiation to the body without hindering cellular and Wi-Fi signals. Similar products are also available for use with laptops, PCs, and tablets. These can be purchased through GIA Wellness or DefenderShield.

The BioInitiative Report

The BioInitiative Report, a study conducted by twenty-nine scientists from all over the world, examined the potential health risks of electromagnetic fields, radiofrequency radiation, and microwave radiation. The report stated, "Chronic exposure to EMFs is associated with increased health risks that vary from impaired learning, headaches, mental confusion, skin rashes, tinnitus, and disorientation to a variety of cancers and neurological diseases like ALS and Alzheimer's." The report identifies as the sources of concern "power lines, cell and cordless phones, cell towers, Wi-Fi, Wi-Max, and wireless Internet."[9]

Smart Technology?

I once believed the more technology, the better. I've changed my mind after learning of the negative effects that constantly emitting devices can have on our health. My research included lectures from medical doctors and scientists whose own health was impacted by this so-called smart technology.

One young engineer who is determined to teach others about the impact of EMFs is Jeromy Johnson. His health went steadily downhill after a multitude of smart meters were installed at his apartment complex below his bedroom window. He soon realized he is EMF-sensitive and is making it his mission to educate others of the potential dangers.[10]

Dr. Libby Darnell, a functional medicine practitioner in Chicago, experienced something similar. Her health mysteriously declined after she moved into a new smart home that integrated all the latest technological bells and whistles. She, too, is educating others in the smarter use of technology.

We must continue researching this topic and using the knowledge we gain to protect our bodies. Of particular concern is the current movement from 4G to 5G technology in our cell phone towers. Dr. Dietrich Klinghardt, founder and chairman of the Institute for Neurobiology in Germany and Switzerland, cautions that these 5G towers will provide *forty times* the impact of the current 4G towers. That's good for faster download speeds and more reliable connections, but perhaps not so good for your body.

Prevention on a Budget

Nearly every home in America is affected by electromagnetic fields. And with the modern proliferation of mobile phones and wireless Internet, possible health issues caused by this technology are reaching crisis levels. My recommendations are:

1. Strongly consider implementing Dr. Davis's recommendations for cell phone use.
2. Limit your exposure to Wi-Fi by going back to computers that are hard wired to the Internet.

3. If your home has Wi-Fi, turn it off during sleeping hours.
4. Remove cordless phones from your home and replace them with hardwired landlines.

In the Cancer Journey

If you are currently battling cancer, I recommend you take the additional steps:

1. Consider buying a cell phone cover or diode that reduces a device's EMF impact on your body.
2. Remove all emitting devices from your bedroom, as these can disrupt sleep in addition to other health concerns.
3. Opt out of allowing a Smart Meter to be placed on your home if it is constantly emitting. Or use technology to shield your family from exposure to the radiation.

Going All Out (For those EMF sensitive)

If anyone in your family is EMF-sensitive and cost is not a major issue, I also recommend that you take the following steps:

1. Hire an EMF consultant to examine your home and make recommendations.
2. Consider moving if your home is located close to a cell phone tower, transmission tower, antenna, etc. You can search for current and future tower sites at www.antennasearch.com.
3. Consider purchasing whole-house EMF protection through a company such as GIA Wellness.

Let's be wise in the use of these new technologies and take precautions to protect our bodies.

STEP EIGHT:

HEALING THE GUT

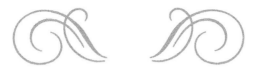

CHAPTER 14

Restoring Your Microbiome

All disease begins in the gut.
—Hippocrates

Death begins in the colon.
—Nobel Prize-winning biologist Eli Metchnikoff

A healthy human body is self-
regulating and self-repairing.
-Dr. Patrick Quillin

Hippocrates, a Greek physician in the fifth century BC, is often called the Father of Medicine. He established medicine as a discipline and profession. He is credited with coining the Hippocratic Oath, and a modified version is still held sacred by physicians today. Currently, we have nearly 10,000 research articles supporting much of what Hippocrates surmised in his detailed medical observations. His analysis of the gut and its role in disease has survived a couple of millennia, leading now to the buzzword of the day in modern medicine: *the microbiome.*

The Microbiome and Immune Health

The microbiome consists of the genetic material of all the microbes (bacteria, fungi, viruses, and other tiny organisms) that live on and in the human body. The human microbiome consists of 10 trillion to 100 trillion symbiotic microbial cells that exist primarily as bacteria in the gut. Your body actually has ten times more microbiota than human cells!

According to Dr. Raphael Kellman, physician of integrative and functional medicine, "The microbiome and immune health are interwoven. It's the microbiome that educates the immune system and connects it to the brain sending messages all over the body like a computer. If our microbiome is restored, our system software is upgraded."[1]

Dr. Tom O'Bryan agrees that the gut is the modulator of brain function. He says, "For every message of the brain going down to the gut, there are nine messages going from the gut to the brain."[2] Dr. Michael Murray refers to the gut as "the central hub to all functions of the body."[3]

We now know what happens in the gut doesn't stay in the gut. In fact, 70-80 percent of the body's immune system cells are located in the upper gastrointestinal tract![4]

None of the body's systems work in isolation. When the gut is healthy, the bacteria in the microbiome help digest food, regulate the immune system, protect against disease-causing bacteria, and produce vitamins that are needed for some of the body's systems to function efficiently. An unhealthy gut allows disease-causing bacteria to accumulate over time and has been linked to such autoimmune disorders as diabetes, rheumatoid arthritis, muscular dystrophy, multiple sclerosis, and fibromyalgia.

Keeping a healthy gut is critical to maintaining balance in the immune system. Kellman cautions, "If our immune system is hypercharged, inflammation results as it fights against our own cells. But when the immune system is too weak, we are more susceptible to diseases such as cancer."[5]

Physician and scientist Dr. Russell Jaffe says, "Our immune systems are constantly defending and repairing. But defense comes first. When defense becomes the preoccupying job of the immune system, repair is deferred."[6]

Each of us needs the immune system to defend and repair to prevent cancer and other diseases. Keeping a healthy microbiome, reducing our toxic load, and getting adequate deep sleep all help the immune system to do both. We must prevent our immune systems from becoming overwhelmed.

The Microbiome, Diabetes, and Cancer

Dr. Brian Mowll, founder of the SweetLife Diabetes Health Centers, says, "Insulin sensitivity is affected by microbiome balance. Diabetes can affect the gut, and the gut can affect insulin resistance." He also believes that leaky gut is closely tied to type 2 diabetes and vascular disease.[7] If you have issues with insulin resistance like me, you need to be proactive by building and sustaining a healthy gut.

The founder of the Institute of Nutritional Endocrinology, Dr. Ritamarie Loscalzo, believes that the microbiome impacts the way estrogens are broken down and eliminated. When they are not properly metabolized, the buildup of these estrogens can contribute to breast and other estrogen-fed cancers.[8]

We tend to think of inflammation in the body as a bad thing, when in fact, inflammation is the immune system's most powerful weapon. On the other hand, *chronic* inflammation can lead to a long list of disorders including arthritis, asthma, atherosclerosis, diabetes, blindness, and yes, cancer. Over time, chronic inflammation can damage DNA and ultimately lead to cancer.[9] It can also promote tumor growth and spread cancer around the body.[10]

A healthy microbiome helps to fight chronic inflammation and lower the risk of cancer.

The Microbiome and Your Emotions

Experience teaches that the microbiome is often affected by negative emotions. When we're upset, our stomach churns. There are cortisol receptors on every immune cell in the lymphoid tissue, and elevated stress causes the body and its immune system to respond. When the gut is out of balance, this creates additional stress on the body, and ongoing stress takes a real toll on the immune system. According to Dr. Joshua Axe, "Gut-friendly bacteria can help manage neurotransmitter activity, which makes them natural antidepressants and anti-anxiety organisms."[11]

Leaky Gut Syndrome

Another buzzword among medical doctors today is a condition called "leaky gut." Leaky gut syndrome is something of a medical mystery, but it's thought to occur when the gut lining becomes chronically inflamed and nutrients are not being absorbed as they should.

Inside the abdominal region, you have an extensive intestinal lining that, when working properly, forms a barrier that controls what gets absorbed into the bloodstream. An unhealthy gut lining may develop large cracks or holes, allowing partially digested food, toxins, and bacteria to leak through your gut lining and eventually find their way into your bloodstream and tissue. This may trigger inflammation and lead to problems within the digestive tract and beyond. "The research world is booming today with studies showing that modifications in the intestinal bacteria and inflammation may play a role in the development of several common chronic diseases."[12]

A new study at Thomas Jefferson University suggests that leaky gut may be at the root of some cancers. "If the intestinal barrier breaks down, it becomes a portal for stuff in the outside world to leak into the inside world," says Dr. Scott Waldman. "When these worlds collide, it can cause many diseases, like inflammation and cancer."[13] This study also suggests that strengthening the intestinal wall could potentially protect people against inflammation and cancer throughout the body. And that's critical information for a cancer patient who is going through chemotherapy.

Dr. O'Bryan calls the gut "the boss" that begins in the mouth and continues through the digestive track to the anus. According to O'Bryan, we generate a new gut lining every three to seven days. He describes the intestines as being lined with shag-carpet-like microvilli that absorb vitamins, minerals, and nutrients. When the layer of shag wears down, problems begin. He also describes holes in this gut wall as tears in cheesecloth that allow even large molecules to penetrate the lining. This gut lining is the most sophisticated and protective one-cell barrier in our body, and we must work to heal tears in the gut. O'Bryan says, "When we are sick, we must ask, 'What's going on in my gut?'"[14]

So how can we heal the gut lining? O'Bryan says, "We must first stop putting fuel on the fire." He encourages his patients to avoid inflammatory foods, processed foods, soft drinks, and fried foods and explore food sensitivities involving wheat, gluten, dairy, etc. We must then rebuild with gut-healing foods. A plant-based diet is great for the gut, as it provides both prebiotic fiber and probiotics. But key to a healthy gut is the diversity of the microbiome. High-intensity exercise will also improve microbiome diversity, which is important for keeping the microbiome healthy and strong.

O'Bryan estimates it can take from six months to several years to rebuild the gut lining. "We simply can't take care of ourselves the way we did ten years ago. Doctors must be trained to look upstream for causes," he urges.[15]

According to Dr. Peter Osborne, best-selling author and a board-certified clinical nutritionist, the biggest threats that cause damage to this gut lining include:

1. Chemicals such as glyphosate, pesticides, herbicides, heavy metals, food preservatives, and dyes
2. Gluten, which can cause gastrointestinal damage
3. Infections, including viral and candida
4. Food sensitivities
5. Medications such as acid reflux medications, antidepressants, pain relievers, and antibiotics[16]

Osborne is just one of many doctors who believe that 70 percent of the human immune system is located in the gut. Leaky gut, a.k.a. intestinal permeability, is the subject of more than 11,000 scientific and medical studies. If we are to be healthy, our digestive tract must serve as a barrier that allows nutrients and other important elements into our bloodstream while keeping bad things out.

Leaky Gut after Chemotherapy

Dr. Axe helped his mother fight lung cancer ten years after her breast cancer and treatment with chemotherapy. After researching the problem, he realized that chemotherapy had destroyed his mother's gut. He immediately began rebuilding her gut with bone broth, high-powered probiotics, L-glutamine powder, coconut oil, blueberries, and raw-culture dairy products.[17] O'Bryan adds to this list stewed apples, root vegetables, fermented foods, and bananas.

Here is Dr. Axe's four-part plan to repair a leaky gut:

1. REMOVE foods and factors that damage the gut.
2. REPLACE with healing foods.
3. REPAIR with specific supplements.
4. REBALANCE with probiotics.[18]

Chemotherapy destroys gut bacteria and the intestinal lining (and therefore the immune system), but many cancer patients and doctors are not being proactive in this area. You can't heal the body if you don't restore the gut once it's been devastated by chemotherapy. After reading extensively about this, I wondered about the condition of my own gut after chemotherapy. I called CTCA to ask what was done to protect this important barrier. I was told that this was the job of the L-glutamine powder and vitamin C infusions I had received.

I am now focusing my attention on adding foods to my diet that will help heal my intestinal gut. My Banana Chocolate Blueberry Smoothie (see chapter 5) is a meal replacement designed for this purpose, and it contains many recommended prebiotic and probiotic ingredients.

Dr. Allan Walker, head of the Harvard Probiotics Symposium and professor at Harvard Medical School, said, "Evidence from clinical research demonstrates that adding good bacteria to the diet promotes a healthy digestive and immune system."[19]

The Doctor Prescribes:

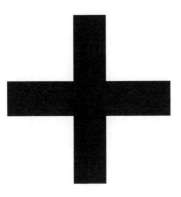

Healing Your Gut

Chemotherapy, like antibiotics, can significantly damage the gut's microbiome. Your gut microbiome is critical to host immunity and response to cancer therapy (especially cancer immunotherapy involving checkpoint inhibitors). It's very important for the cancer patient to take a good probiotic daily and eat only foods that promote a healthy gut. Immunotherapies don't generally work as well unless the patient is using a good probiotic.

Dr. Robert L. Elliott

Glyphosate and the Gut

Glyphosate, an herbicide heavily used on GMOs and other crops, is an irritant to the gut lining. Dr. Osborne identifies it as one of the major culprits causing damage to the gut lining of Americans. Many others have also expressed concerns about glyphosate, including Dr. Dan Pompa, who himself overcame neurotoxic illness and heavy metal poisoning. Pompa believes, "When glyphosate enters our bodies through our gut, it shuts down a major detox pathway and opens up the blood-brain barrier."[20]

Dr. Stephanie Seneff, senior researcher at Massachusetts Institute of Technology who has spent much of her life's work researching glyphosate, agrees and adds, "Glyphosate kills bacteria in the gut and tears through the gut lining," resulting in inflammation in the body.[21] As we have seen, chronic inflammation can damage DNA and ultimately lead to any number of serious health conditions, including cancer.

Conversely, the same company that told us DDT, PCBs, and Agent Orange were safe is now declaring that glyphosate is perfectly safe. This company, Monsanto, has an inordinate amount of control over the safety of Americans' food. In 1987, the U.S. was using 11 million pounds of Roundup, a popular Monsanto product that contains glyphosate. Today we use nearly 300 million pounds annually.[22]

Honestly, there exists conflicting evidence. Some see Monsanto as a good fairy who helps the world food supply. But others see them as the Wicked Witch of the Midwest. Monsanto's research declares that Roundup is harmless, while other research clearly shows serious issues. What's a sensible person to believe? More and more people are going to great lengths to avoid glyphosate and other pesticides and herbicides. I'm not waiting until the evidence becomes overwhelming, especially since high levels of glyphosate and other pesticides were discovered in my body.

Some days I wonder why the EPA, USDA, and FDA aren't on the same page as their counterparts in other countries? Why does the World Health Organization's International Agency for Research on Cancer (IARC) classify glyphosate as "probably carcinogenic to humans" when the EPA, USDA, and FDA do not?[23] Why can't the agencies that are supposed to protect us connect the dots between the rising incidents of chronic disease and the rising use of chemicals in our foods? Why have more than half the countries in Europe acted to ban GMO foods[24] when the U.S. won't act to even *label* them?

The IARC's finding motivated more than one million people in the European Union to ask for a moratorium on glyphosate. French president Emmanuel Macron has vowed to ban glyphosate in France within the next three years.[25]

California's Proposition 65, which passed in 1986, alerted consumers to chemicals that may cause cancer. In 2017, glyphosate was added to the list of chemicals that California believes to be carcinogenic. The mandate requires a warning label on all products containing glyphosate stating, "Ingredients are known to the state of California to cause cancer and birth defects and other reproductive harm."[26] School districts in Burbank, Irvine, and Glendale have banned glyphosate from their properties.

In 2018, a California jury found Monsanto liable in a lawsuit filed by a school groundskeeper who claimed the company's glyphosate-based weed killers caused his cancer. He was awarded $289 million in damages. The jury found that Monsanto had failed to warn the plaintiff and other consumers of the cancer risks posed by its weed killers.[27] Brett Wisner, the attorney who represented the plaintiff, said, "Monsanto has specifically gone out of its way to bully . . . and to fight independent researchers." Wisner presented information showing that Monsanto also rejected critical research and expert warnings over the years while pursuing only favorable analyses of their products.[28]

Monsanto, which was recently acquired by Bayer AG, faces more than 8,000 similar lawsuits across the U.S.[29] The company appealed the verdict and declared that its weed killers do not cause cancer. The appeal lowered the damages to $78 million. Since then, more trials and verdicts against Monsanto have occurred.

Self-Protection Is the Best Policy

I've learned not to depend on our government to protect me. I'm the only one who can proactively take measures to protect my body from the toxic world we live in. With Monsanto's unreliable history involving chemicals such as Agent Orange and funding of research that only supports their causes, I choose to follow the money on this one—and it leads to the pockets of many politicians. Politicians and consumers alike must be educated regarding the known facts about glyphosate and other pesticides.

Our country is inundated with fake foods. It's important to eat real, live food as God made it. Many are calling GMO foods "God Move Over" foods. Only you can decide if glyphosate is for you or against you. I urge you to do your homework before making a decision.

After surviving all the cancer treatments and surgeries, my husband and I celebrated with a river cruise through the heart of Europe. I called the cruise chef before leaving to inquire about the chemicals in the food. I was delighted to discover that the countries we'd be passing through were among those banning GMO foods. After two weeks on the cruise, my gut was happy and thriving.

Paul's Advice to Timothy

In his first letter to Timothy, the apostle Paul wrote, "No longer drink only water, but use a little wine for your stomach's sake and your frequent infirmities" (1 Timothy 5:23). Paul's advice to his protégé has caused much controversy within the modern church. Those in favor of drinking wine often see it as permission to drink any kind of alcohol. Others wish Paul had never given this bit of advice.

If you've traveled in a developing country where you consumed contaminated water, your understanding of this verse becomes clearer. This happened to my dad and me while traveling in Romania on a mission trip. After discovering our "bottled water" was really empty bottles refilled with tap water, we knew we were in for a rough plane ride home.

Our trip leader, John Simmons, who was always prepared, gave us two options: 1) We could take a strong antibiotic for ten days or 2) we could have a glass of wine with dinner. Those members of the group who took neither the antibiotic nor the wine suffered greatly. I knew even then that it's best to take an antibiotic only when absolutely necessary. Dad and I decided to try the wine as medicine, and it worked.

While touring the castles and cathedrals of Europe, Alton and I learned that the making of wine was a necessity throughout much of history. Clean drinking water was scarce, and watered-down wine was a safer alternative.

Research now shows that drinking red wine significantly increases levels of bacteria called bifidobacteria. These bacteria reduce gut wall permeability and also lead to lower levels of inflammation.[30]

A study by the *Journal of American Nutrition* found that red wine (made with or without alcohol) produced improvements in the bacterial composition of the gut, lowered blood pressure, and reduced levels of a protein associated with inflammation.[31]

Red wine is also known for containing polyphenols, which are natural antioxidants, and small amounts of resveratrol, which also reduces inflammation.[32]

Note that the apostle Paul said "a little wine." Moderation is key. However, you don't have to drink wine to get these same benefits. Red grapes and blueberries are high in both antioxidants and resveratrol.

Prevention on a Budget

A healthy gut is critical to maintaining a healthy immune system, which is needed to both defend and repair the human body. Our gut health and microbiome is largely influenced by our diet. My recommendations are:

1. Eat 10–13 servings of fruits and vegetables daily. These provide prebiotic fiber, phytochemicals, and nutrients that build and repair the gut lining.
2. Eat two to three serving per day of probiotic foods such as fermented vegetables, kefir, apple cider vinegar, kombucha tea, and yogurt.
3. Avoid the use of antibiotics unless absolutely necessary. After completing a course of antibiotics, actively use foods to repair your gut lining and replace good bacteria that was lost to the meds.
4. Eliminate from your diet foods that you are sensitive to and those that cause damage to the gut lining.

In the Cancer Journey

If you are currently battling cancer, also do the following:

1. Use L-Glutamine powder after each chemotherapy treatment to protect the gut wall. CTCA recommended to me ten grams of this powder three times a day in a liquid for five days after chemotherapy.
2. Take a diverse probiotic containing many strains of bacteria daily.
3. Drink smoothies similar to the one I describe in chapter 5. This helped to rebuild my immune system and restore the gut lining.

Going All Out

If you have the material means, also do the following:

1. Consider taking vitamin C infusions twenty-four hours before chemotherapy to build your immune system and protect the gut. Let your oncologist know if you are getting these infusions.

Unfortunately, a healthy gut was a preventative step I discovered *after* my treatments, but I'm celebrating that I learned of it in time to work on it following chemotherapy. Protecting and restoring my gut prevented more health issues down the road.

Remember, fruits and vegetables are key to the health of your gut and microbiome. As Dorothy learned, fruits and vegetables are found all along the Yellow Brick Road. Just be careful as to their source. In this day of GMOs, it's probably not wise to pick your apples from a talking tree.

IF YOU'RE ON THE PINK BRICK ROAD...

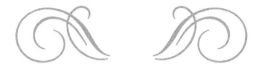

CHAPTER 15

For Breast and Estrogen-Fed Cancer Only

*Our soul waits for the LORD; He is our help and our
shield. For our heart shall rejoice in Him, because
we have trusted in His holy name. Let Your mercy,
O LORD, be upon us, just as we hope in You.*
—Psalm 33:20–22

According to the World Health Organization, breast cancer is the most commonly diagnosed cancer in women worldwide. In America, an estimated 252,710 women will be diagnosed each year, and more than 40,500 will die. This makes breast cancer the second-leading cause of death among women in the U.S., behind heart disease. What's even more astounding is that about 85 percent of breast cancers occur in women who have no family history of it.[1]

Breast Cancer and Genetics

The most common cause of hereditary breast cancer is an inherited mutation in the BRCA1 and BRCA2 genes. In normal cells, these genes help prevent cancer by producing proteins that keep the cells from growing abnormally. Mutated versions of these genes cannot stop abnormal growth, however, and that leads to cancer.

If you inherited a mutated copy of either gene from a parent, you have a higher risk of breast cancer. In some families with BRCA1 mutations, the lifetime risk of breast cancer is as high as 80 percent, whereas on average the risk seems to be in the range of 55-65 percent for those who are carriers of the gene. For BRCA2 mutations the risk is lower, around 45 percent.

In my case, genetic testing showed that I did not have any genes related to breast cancer. Having one of these genes is an automatic mastectomy in many doctors' eyes. Some doctors and integrative practitioners believe that making lifestyle changes can trump genetic expression. But for many, the surgery is worth the peace of mind.

Living in an Estrogenic World

I was shocked to learn I had been diagnosed with estrogen-fed breast cancer. I was not taking estrogen hormones, nor was I knowingly eating foods that contained estrogen. And I'd never taken birth control pills. I was subsequently diagnosed post-menopausal when my estrogen levels were minimal. Nevertheless, I had joined the estrogen-fed club along with 80 percent of breast cancer patients. (NOTE: Ovarian, endometrial, and uterine cancers can also be estrogen-fed.)

So, what had happened?

My answer finally came when Canadian cancer coach Alicia Mazari told me at a medical convention, "Ginny, we live in an estrogenic world." At first, I wondered what world she was living in, but I later discovered that she was right, and *I* was the sleepwalker who needed to wake up and recognize the toxic world around me.

I learned about xenoestrogens, which are synthetic chemical compounds that mimic the effects of estrogen and interact with cellular receptor sites. These chemicals are also endocrine disruptors—they lodge in fat cells and work synergistically when combined with other hormone disruptors, causing major problems at the cellular level.[2]

Xenoestrogens can be found in a variety of everyday items, including plastic water bottles, Styrofoam products, cosmetics, nail polish, cleaning products, the lining of canned foods, and fruits and vegetables sprayed with pesticides, as well as chicken, beef, and dairy products from animals raised on certain kinds of feed.

Practitioners of integrative medicine recommend limiting exposure to xenoestrogens as much as possible. Choosing hormone-free dairy and animal products and organic produce is a good place to start, along with removing from your home things that have an estrogenic-like effect on the body.

Another suggestion is to remove or limit your alcohol intake. Alcohol is believed to increase a woman's cancer risk because it increases levels of estrogen and other hormones associated with hormone-receptor-positive breast cancer. According to Dr. Robert Pendergrast, "Alcohol increases cancer risk, and specifically increases breast cancer risk because it increases aromatase activity."[3]

A 1996 analysis of epidemiologic data from more than fifty studies worldwide found that women who were current or recent users of birth control pills had a slightly higher risk of developing breast cancer than women who had never used the pill. The risk was highest for women who started using oral contraceptives as teenagers.[4]

Among men who have been diagnosed with breast cancer, 90 percent of these cancers are estrogen-driven. This is even more evidence that we live in an estrogenic world. Men can get breast cancer even though their bodies produce only small amounts of estrogen. As with female breast cancer, it's often not just the natural estrogen causing the cancer, but possibly the presence of xenoestrogens that mimic estrogen coming from the outside into the body.[5] It's time we all wake up.

Estrogens—the Weak, the Bad, and the Good

Estrogen, known as the "female hormone," consists of three different types that are naturally produced in the body. These three types are:

Estrone (E1)
Estrone is produced mainly in the liver and fat cells. It's the "weak" form of estrogen, and the main one produced during menopause. It can be converted into estradiol, the more aggressive estrogen.

Estradiol (E2)

Estradiol is produced in the ovaries. It is the main form of estrogen produced during the reproductive years. Estradiol plays a major role in giving us energy, sleep, sexual drive, healthy bones and skin, and *moisturizing* the gut lining, eyes, and vagina. Unfortunately, estradiol is a strong growth stimulator, and elevated levels are linked to higher risks of female cancer. Although it serves many important functions, it's sometimes referred to as the "bad estrogen."

Estriol (E3)

Estriol is made in the liver and breast cells and by the placenta during pregnancy. It's sometimes referred to as the "good estrogen" due to its highly protective effect[6] of reducing the more aggressive estradiol and protecting against radiation-induced cancer of the breast.[7]

These three forms of estrogen work together and are an important part of a woman's well-being. Estrogen circulates in the blood, passes easily in and out of all organs and tissues, and is eventually metabolized by enzymes in the liver and excreted through the kidneys. Dr. Henry Lemon developed a "normal" ratio for these estrogens that is referred to in hormone testing. If your ratio of more aggressive estrogens, E1 and E2, are higher than the less aggressive and protective estrogen, E3, then your chances of developing an estrogen-fed breast cancer increases.[8]

According to Dr. Veronique Desaulniers, another step to understanding your hormone balance and risk for cancer is to determine if you are metabolizing or breaking down estrogen properly.[9] If these estrogens are not properly metabolized, they can be recirculated in the body. Dr. Pendergrast believes body fat percentage and the accumulation of estrogen over time both increase a woman's risk for breast cancer.[10]

Estrogen is highest during puberty and pregnancy, yet I was well beyond these stages of life. It took me a while to realize that my estrogen dominance was originating from the accumulation of natural estrogens and from the addition of xenoestrogens entering my body from outside sources.

The Doctor Prescribes:

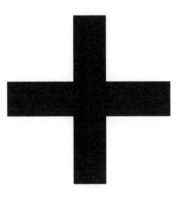

Prioritizing Your Health

Breast cancer patients should wait to have breast reconstruction done until after they receive the results from the sentinel node biopsy. Many plastic surgeons rush the reconstruction at the time of primary surgery, before the test results are known. I understand that saving the breast is the preferred method for the self-esteem of the woman, but sometimes it is best to remove the breast for the health of the patient. It is unwise to put cosmetic concerns before treatment of the disease.

Dr. Robert L. Elliott

The Bear of a Pill

There are several reproductive cancers that can be driven by estrogen, including ovarian, cervical, breast, and uterine (endometrial). Unfortunately, aromatase inhibitors (which stop the production of estrogen in postmenopausal women by blocking the enzyme aromatase) can wreak havoc on your body. But they can be powerful for sending cancer into remission. This pill alone temporarily reversed my mom's metastatic cancer. My oncologist told me that this pill lowered my chances of recurrence by 40 percent! For premenopausal women, Tamoxifen is usually prescribed.

Due to *unbearable* side effects, many women walk away from the anti-hormone therapies recommended by their oncologists. I understand, and don't think I didn't consider it. After five months of taking Femara, my sleepless nights had increased, my brain fog had become unbearable, and my bones and joints ached. I remember panicking the day I found I was unable to get out of my chair. I have to be able to sleep, think, and move! After I told my doctor, he switched me to a pill called Anastrozole (generic for Arimidex). It appears to be doing the job with lesser side effects.

Estrogen is not essential for life, but it does contribute to one's quality of life. I was disheartened when I realized my journey wouldn't be over after the chemotherapy and Herceptin infusions. It would continue for five years from the time I began taking "this little pill." Some doctors even recommend taking the pills for anywhere from ten years to life. No, thanks.

Below are the remedies I learned to deal with the side effects of this pill. There are also natural ways that a woman can reduce estrogen dominance when her five- to ten-year anti-hormone therapies have ended, or if she has chosen not to take the pill.

Remedies for the Side Effects of Aromatase Inhibitors

Today, some insurance companies are offering to provide aromatase inhibitors for menopausal women in an effort to lessen their risk for estrogen-fed cancers. I don't recommend taking them unless you are considered high-risk or already have an estrogen-fed cancer. Listed below are the remedies for dealing with "the bear":

Hot flashes: Take 1000 mg of primrose oil daily.

Bone and Joint Pain: Exercise and use bone broth protein with collagen in smoothies.

Brain Fog: Exercise and use a few drops of peppermint oil and rosemary oil in your shampoo to stimulate brain circulation. Take krill oil or omega-3 supplements for brain function.

Loss of Bone Density: Use daily weight-bearing exercises and yoga to apply pressure to the osteoblasts to produce new bone. Eat greens alone or in smoothies to supply calcium and minerals.

Depression: Exercise daily to increase chemicals in the brain that elevate mood.

Hair Loss: Add a few drops of rosemary oil to your shampoo.

Insomnia: Use natural compounds from the plant world.

If you change your lifestyle habits as recommended in the eight steps discussed in this book, your cancer is less likely to return. If your cancer does not return, your doctor will likely stop your estrogen-blocking or reducing medication after five years. Then your body can rebuild and recover. But you must also look at ways to decrease your own estrogen dominance for future prevention.

Decreasing Estrogen Dominance

OB-GYN Dr. Christiane Northrup offers the following ways to decrease estrogen dominance in your body:

- Add fiber to your diet (2 Tablespoons of ground flax seeds daily). This helps estrogen to be removed by the large intestine. If stool remains in the bowel too long, estrogen can recirculate and create estrogen dominance.
- Eat a healthy diet of fresh fruit and vegetables, healthy fats, and good proteins.
- Take a good vitamin-mineral supplement made from whole foods (not synthetic).
- Cleanse the liver. "When the liver has to work hard to eliminate toxins, such as alcohol, drugs, caffeine, and environmental agents, the liver's capacity to cleanse the blood of estrogen is compromised," says Dr. Northrup.
- Reduce stress (see chapter 9). Stress causes cortisol levels to go up, and estrogen follows. [11]

Adequate sleep, exercise, hydration, proper nutrition, and lowering your toxic load will all help the liver to work at optimum capacity—the way God intended.

Dr. Joshua Axe also recommends keeping insulin levels low with estrogen-fed cancers and estrogen dominance. High blood sugar also causes estrogen levels to escalate. Remember, breasts are made from fat tissue, and we store toxins in our fat tissue.

Emotions and Breast Cancer

A woman's breasts give nourishment to her babies, pleasure to her spouse, and confirm her sexual identity. This makes breast cancer an emotional issue for many. This is why surgeons today are making every effort to save a woman's breasts if possible.

Nursing your baby provides the best possible nutrients for your child while also lowering your risk for breast cancer. That's because breastfeeding inhibits the production of estrogen by the ovaries, which decreases a woman's overall lifetime estrogen exposure. [12]

Sugar and Breast Cancer Risk

Dietary sugar has been shown to increase the risk of breast cancer tumors and metastasis to the lungs. MD Anderson Cancer Center published a 2016 study finding that high amounts of dietary sugar in the typical Western diet seem to affect an enzymatic signaling pathway known as 12-LOX (12-lipoxygenase) in a way that increases breast cancer risk. Dr. Peiying Yang summarizes the study results:

> We found that sucrose intake in mice comparable to levels of Western diets led to increased tumor growth and metastasis, when compared to a non-sugar starch diet. . . . Prior research has examined the role of sugar, especially glucose, and energy-based metabolic pathways in cancer development. However, the inflammatory cascade may be an alternative route of studying sugar-driven carcinogenesis that warrants further study.[13]

Flaxseed and DIM to the Rescue

Sayer Ji of Green Med Info believes that flaxseed's role in fighting breast cancer is one of the more compelling areas of research. He says, "Flaxseed has an exceptional nutritional profile, and it is a medicinal powerhouse."[14]

A study published in 2005 in the *Clinical Cancer Research* journal involved patients who received a 25-gram flaxseed-containing muffin over the course of thirty-two days. After observing a reduction in tumor markers and an increase in apoptosis in the flaxseed-treated patients, the authors concluded, "Dietary flaxseed has the potential to reduce tumor growth in patients with breast cancer."[15]

Sayer Ji points to flaxseed's phytoestrogen compounds, which may interact with estrogen receptors and prevent and/or regress hormone-associated cancers. Although some in the medical field view phytoestrogens as something to avoid, this research indicates otherwise. Dr. Axe and Dr. Colbert both contend that the lignans in flaxseed can block activity of the enzyme that converts other hormones into estrogen.

Dr. Desaulniers was the first medically trained individual to answer the question that plagued me, "How did I get an estrogen-fed cancer?" Her explanation is powerful:

> Zeno or chemical estrogens are everywhere. Many are coming into our bodies through food, water, and the air we breathe. When the liver can't methylate these excessive estrogens into healthy metabolites to urinate them out of the body, these aggressive estrogens keep circulating and build up in our bodies.

When I first heard her say this at The Truth About Cancer conference in Dallas in October 2016, I said, "Now *that* makes sense." She also recommends limiting exposure to these estrogens, keeping the liver working properly, detoxing the body, testing to determine if methylation is happening properly in the liver, and using flaxseeds to prevent estrogen-fed cancers.

Dr. Kenna Barber, my naturopathic doctor at CTCA Newnan, explained this to me even further when she recommended that I consider taking a DIM (diindolylmethane) supplement:

> DIM, which is extracted from cruciferous vegetables, helps shunt the majority of estrogen metabolism in the liver through a healthy, benign pathway. The liver is responsible for metabolizing estrogens, and it has one of two pathways to choose from—one pathway creates benign metabolites that do not stimulate estrogen receptors, and the other pathway creates metabolites that can stimulate estrogen receptors.

> Anytime there is an estrogen-positive (sensitive) cancer, one wants to minimize the amount of estrogens and metabolites that can stimulate the estrogen receptors of the cancer. DIM helps do that by supporting the liver to primarily use the metabolic pathway that will not produce stimulatory metabolites. DIM therefore, becomes 'anti-cancerous' for estrogenic-based cancers.

Then she zeroed in on the value of flaxseeds for an estrogen-fed cancer patient:

Flaxseeds are phytoestrogens. Phytoestrogens can act like estrogen in the body, but in a weaker way. They can attach to and stimulate estrogen receptors, but they do so in a more protective fashion. Phytoestrogens in limited amounts attach to estrogen receptors, preventing stronger, more stimulating estrogens from being able to attach to those same receptors.

An average of two tablespoons of ground flaxseeds daily is a safe amount for those with estrogen-positive cancers. Flaxseed as a lignan has also been shown to reduce the more active forms of estrogen in post-menopausal women. Therefore, in limited doses, flaxseed can be protective even with estrogen-receptor positive cancers.

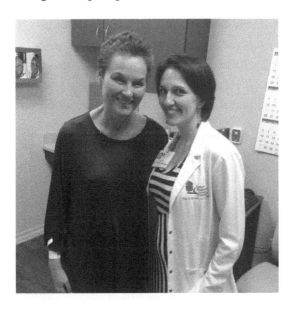

Dr. Kenna Barber, my naturopathic doctor, has
been an important asset in my journey.

I always like to get opinions backed by research on any topic from at least five medically trained experts before I apply it to my life. Dr. Connie Ross, my former integrative medical doctor, began promoting the lignans in flaxseeds as prevention for breast cancer years ago. I've just shared seven opinions from experts whom I respect. I wish I had listened sooner, but I didn't see myself as being at high risk for this type of cancer. Please hear me: *We are all high risk for estrogen-fed cancers in this culture!*

Other Anti-Estrogenic Foods

According to Dr. Jockers, anti-inflammatory foods that are rich in saturated and omega-3 fatty acids—including 100 percent organic, grass-fed beef and dairy, organic poultry, wild-caught salmon, and wild game—are anti-estrogenic. Plant-based fats such as avocados, coconut oil, and olive oil are powerful anti-estrogenic superfoods. Raw nuts and seeds such as almonds, pecans, walnuts, chia, pumpkin, and hemp seeds are also rich in anti-estrogenic plant sterols.[16]

Jockers also recommends consuming organic acids to enhance the body's ability to remove unwanted estrogenic molecules. Organic acids include freshly squeezed lemons (which are rich in citric acid), apple cider vinegar (which contains acetic acid), and fermented raw dairy (which contains lactic acid) from grass-fed cows. These are great for enhancing detoxification processes and neutralizing bad estrogen metabolites.[17]

The Missing Ingredient in Our Diet

According to author Dr. David Brownstein, "Every cell in your body needs iodine." He believes that iodine deficiency is the main cause behind the epidemic of thyroid problems in America. In his practice, Brownstein has found that nearly 95 percent of his patients have an iodine deficiency. The thyroid gland needs sufficient iodine to produce the thyroid hormone, which is important to your overall health. Today, Synthroid is one of the most prescribed drugs on the market.

Brownstein believes iodine deficiency is also fueling the rise in breast and prostate cancers. He recommends 6 to 50 mg of iodine per day for restoring healthy levels. Dr. Ross recommended that I take a kelp supplement for prevention, but check with your doctor for his or her recommendation. Your thyroid must be working properly!

Brownstein points to a wealth of research showing the connection between iodine deficiency and breast cancer. He believes that iodine deficiency is a causative factor in breast cancer and fibrocystic disease. He sees the breasts as one of the body's main storage and utilization sites for iodine and feels iodine is necessary for the maintenance of normal breast tissue.[18] He says, "Iodine deficiency causes estrogen production to increase, and it also leads to an increased sensitivity of breast tissue to estrogen."[19]

The Hippies Were Right!

Yes, the hippies were right about a few things in the 1960s and early '70s, though clearly not everything. Remember the days of free love and burning bras? Free love caused many problems in the long run. Evidence, however, is emerging from around the world showing that wearing bras that are too constrictive and made with toxic chemicals in the fabric may be another cause contributing to the rise in breast cancer.

The research came to light in 1995, when Sydney Singer and wife Soma Grismaije published the book *Dressed to Kill*. As applied medical anthropologists, they studied how our culture is making us sick. After Soma found a lump in her breast, they began to research the link between bras and breast cancer.

As Sydney helped his wife to unfasten her bra, he noticed red marks where her bra was restricting the flow of her lymphatic system. He reasoned intuitively, "If one constricts the breast, the draining of the lymphatic system gets cut off." This in turn restricts the removal of toxins in the breast which must be flushed out by the lymphatic system.

Actually, this couple was not the first to raise questions regarding the connection between bras and breast cancer. Dr. William John Mayo, one of the founders of the Mayo Clinic, wrote an article, "Susceptibility to Cancer," published in the 1931 *Annals of Surgery*. Mayo wrote, "Cancer of the breast occurs largely among civilized women. In those countries where breasts are allowed to be exposed, that is, not compressed or irritated by clothing, it is rare." He went on to say:

The problem caused by bras is due to their constriction of the breasts, particularly of the lymphatic system, which is responsible for eliminating toxins, cancer cells, bacteria, viruses, and cellular debris from the breasts. The lymphatics are an essential circulatory pathway of the immune system. Constrict the microscopic, easily compressed lymph vessels with tight bras, and the result is lymph fluid congestion in the breasts, or lymph stasis, along with tissue toxification. This can cause breast pain and cysts (which are filled with this lymph fluid). Over time, as the breasts progressively become toxic from impaired lymphatic drainage, cancer could result.[20]

Now, I'm not advocating exposing your breasts. I'm advocating lessening the constriction and hours of wearing a bra. We've all also seen pictures of women with sagging breasts; some support may be needed.

Although Sydney and Soma faced much opposition from the bra industry and no support from the ACS, research from around the world is beginning to support their claims. A study done in Brazil in 2016 reveals that wearing a tight bra for many hours a day is associated with increased risk of breast cancer.[21]

While visiting my doctors at CTCA in Newnan, Georgia, I mentioned what I'd learned. One doctor's response was telling. "What's the name of that book again?" he asked. "I must admit it makes sense. I'd like to look more into this."

Sydney and Soma made the following recommendations:

- Wear the correct size of bra, one that does not constrict your breasts or leave red marks when you remove it.
- Purchase bras made of organic materials instead of materials containing chemicals. Otherwise, when you sweat, it's like your breasts are being marinated in toxins.
- Avoid plastic or metal underwires and push-up bras that lift your breasts in an unnatural way. (Since husbands love these bras, occasional use is okay.)

- When you wear a bra, limit the wearing to less than twelve hours in a day. Don't sleep in a bra.
- Consider going braless for one month to allow your breasts to decompress and the circulation to work normally.[22]

This information encouraged me to change my undergarments and nighties to 100 percent cotton. I decided that anything I wear that close to my body must be natural fibers that breathe and don't contain toxins. And I don't wear constricting bras.

Early Detection Is Key

John Hopkins Medical Center reports that 40 percent of breast cancer patients first discover the tumor themselves. This information should encourage you to self-monitor your breasts monthly in addition to getting yearly mammograms. I can't emphasize this enough. I found my own lump four months after my yearly checkup and six months after a mammogram detected nothing. If I had waited six more months with an aggressive cancer, I might not be here today. *Don't underestimate self-checks.*

In addition to the semiannual mammograms required by CTCA, I also get one thermogram and one ultrasound done by HerScan. This way, I am checked every three months. I also do a vitamin C infusion after each mammogram to reduce the radiation buildup. The thermogram and ultrasound do not involve radiation.

The new 3D mammogram (which involves no more radiation than flying across the US in a plane) is a blessing for those of us who have dense breasts. Twenty-eight states now have laws that require mammography centers to inform women with dense breast tissue (about 40-50 percent of us) that it may increase the risk of cancer and obscure a malignancy on a mammogram.[23] Ask your doctor if you have dense breasts.

Two mammograms missed my cancer. If you have dense breasts, find a breast-imaging center with this updated technology even if you must travel to find one.

The Doctor Prescribes:

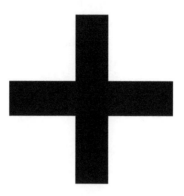

Don't Fear the Mammogram

Many women still fear that mammograms put out too much radiation to be safe. This is not true. Today's equipment uses lower doses of radiation to produce high-quality images, using technology that has been available for almost thirty years. The benefits of mammography far outweigh the possible harm from the minimal radiation exposure.

Dr. Robert L. Elliott

American Cancer Society Reduces Number of Mammograms

In October 2015, the American Cancer Society announced new screening guidelines that surprisingly reduced the number of mammograms recommended for women. The ACS now recommends that women wait until age 45 to begin having mammograms, and continue annually until age 54. After age 54, they recommend women continue them every other year. High-risk women may begin earlier than age 45.

Keep in mind that mammograms can have false positives and sometimes miss tumors. To make up for these limitations, breastcancer.org agrees that breast self-examination and regular breast examinations by an experienced healthcare professional are needed.[24]

Some women may choose regular self-examination and thermograms yearly, or alternate by having a mammogram one year and a thermogram the next.

My Recommendations for Preventing Estrogen-Fed Cancer and Recurrence

According to the CDC, breast cancer is the most common cause of cancer-related death among Hispanic women and the second-most common among white, black, Asian/Pacific islanders, and Native American women. We simply cannot afford to ignore the danger. Here then are my recommendations:

1. Use 1–2 tablespoons of freshly ground flaxseed as fiber daily (can be in smoothie) and always hydrate properly.
2. Keep vitamin D3 levels in the 70–90 ng/ml range.
3. Use a kelp or iodine supplement to keep your thyroid working properly.
4. Self-check your breasts monthly.
5. Schedule yearly medical screenings: mammogram, thermogram, or HerScan ultrasound, or alternate.
6. Avoid using plastic bottles, cans lined with estrogen, and dairy and meat products containing estrogen and xenoestrogens.

7. Eat organic fruits and vegetables unless one of the Clean Fifteen.
8. Replace common body care products with coconut oil and products made without chemicals and hormone disruptors.
9. Monitor your blood sugar levels. Your A1C should be below 5.7.
10. Exercise and monitor your body weight and stress levels.
11. Consider wearing a non-constricting sports bra made from natural fibers, thus allowing your breasts to breathe. Avoid sleeping in your bra at night. Limit the time you wear a bra to no more than 12 hours per day.
12. Increase your intake of cruciferous vegetables daily or use diindolylmethane (DIM) to help your body neutralize reactive estrogen metabolites.
13. Consider drinking my Banana Chocolate Blueberry Smoothie or a variation that contains 2 cups of cruciferous vegetables and ground flax seeds.
14. Jumpstart your day with my daily detox drink.
15. Exercise daily to keep your lymphatic system working properly.
16. If you have dense breasts, insist on a 3D mammogram or ultrasound.

For those on the cancer journey dealing with breast cancer or other estrogen-fed cancer, you must consider how you will continue to reduce the estrogen dominance in your body once your doctor says you can stop taking the aromatase inhibitor. You need to address the root cause and learn how to prevent recurrence.

Dorothy knew that tornadoes were common in Kansas. So, when the winds began to pick up and the signs pointed to danger, she should have taken shelter sooner. She was distracted by her dog until her chances for survival were nearly gone with the wind. Breast cancer has become far too common for you to ignore the danger any longer.

If you desire to prevent breast cancer, you *must* seek to lower the estrogens in your body. Realize that you could be the one in eight and put a prevention plan in place now. Using common sense gives us hope for the future.

DESTINATION:
EMERALD CITY

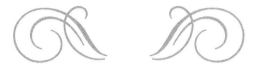

CHAPTER 16

Promoting Longevity while Anticipating Heaven

It is good for me that I have been afflicted,
that I may learn Your statutes.
—Psalm 119:71

The doctor of the future will give no medicine, but will
interest his patients in the care of the human frame,
in diet and in the cause and prevention of disease.
—Thomas A. Edison

The biblical Adam lived to be 930 years old. Noah's grandfather Methuselah would live to the ripe old age of 969. But "the wickedness of man was great in the earth" (Genesis 6:6), and about the time of the Great Flood, God chose to limit a person's time on the earth to no more than 120 years (Genesis 6:3).

Moses was the greatest prophet in the Old Testament. It's interesting that he lived exactly 120 years and was not feeble or ailing (Deuteronomy 34:7). When Moses' work on the earth was complete, God took him home.

My cancer journey causes me to wonder, how many of us will live to completely fulfill God's purpose in our lives? How many will cut out early on our life's purpose because of our poor eating habits and foolish lifestyle?

Modern medicine offers numerous breakthrough technologies

including the finest diagnostic instruments, emergency procedures, and life-saving surgeries ever known to man. And yet chronic disease is on the rise in part because we so often overlook the role of nutrition and lifestyle choices that could prevent many chronic conditions in the first place.

When symptoms arise, we simply run to the doctor and say, "Fix this. Use a pill if you can, surgery if you must." We expect a one-time prescription to remedy ills we've spent a lifetime of bad choices working toward. The good news is, we can prevent and/or heal so many chronic conditions ourselves with a series of lifestyle changes involving hydration, regular rest, daily exercise, and a radical shift in diet.

Paradigm Shift toward Prevention

Instead of expecting your doctor (or wizard) to fix everything, take a proactive approach to your health. Make prevention your goal and ask, *What can I do to prevent disease? What can I do to take care of this God–given temple?*

If you have been diagnosed with cancer, here are the prime questions you should be asking:

- Did I do anything that contributed to my diagnosis? Is there something in my home, workplace, diet, activity level, or other lifestyle choices that may have caused my cancer?
- How can I assist my doctor in fighting the cancer?
- What steps can I implement now to enable my body to work optimally during treatments?
- What can I do to prevent recurrence of the cancer?

In this life, we will all face trials, even those of us who are God's children. Some of these trials will occur by chance, some will arise by the hand of others, and some are simply "my bad" scenarios (the consequences of our own actions).

It's true that I'm not responsible for the rise of processed foods and GMOs, the increased levels of toxic chemicals in everyday items, or for the mercury amalgam fillings that were placed in my mouth. (Admittedly, the cavities were my fault.) However, I *can* make better choices by eating organic foods, joining a food co-op, or growing my own fruits and vegetables. I can filter my water, reduce my dependence on household chemicals, and eliminate some toxins by replacing dangerous cosmetics and personal care products with safer alternatives. I can gradually replace those mercury amalgam fillings with ceramic fillings. I can also implement daily and biannual detox programs to lower my toxic load and reduce the chemicals and metals in my body.

I must honestly look at the "my bads." I was not proactive in dealing with the grief that dominated my life for fifteen years as all four of our parents passed. Nor did I pay any attention to my gut lining or plan my meals using food as medicine. I was blissfully ignorant of all the toxins accumulating in my body. Awareness is important, and ignorance is not an excuse.

Oh, the lessons I've learned!

I am what I eat.

I am what I eat "eats."

I am what my body can't digest or eliminate.

My emotions also have a powerful effect on my body.

My body is a temple, and God commands me to care for and nourish it.

The body's God-given ability to heal is miraculous.

The Power of the Eight Steps

Whether you have been diagnosed with cancer or you purchased this book because you're determined to prevent cancer (or a recurrence), the eight steps to health that we've discussed in this book are more than just a good idea. Inasmuch as it depends on you, a healthy body is important to achieve your fullest, God-given potential. Of course, you can't control some diseases, accidents, or your genetics. But you *can* make wise choices that reduce your health risks and allow your body's immune system to function as designed by God. Let's review the eight steps.

In the first place, there is an element of dehydration in every illness. If you want your body to work as God designed it, you must adequately hydrate. The chemical reactions in each of your body's systems and every cell must have an ample supply of clean water to function properly.

Second, your body requires deep sleep to recharge and repair itself and defend against disease, including cancer. Inadequate sleep reduces the body's production of the cancer-fighting hormone melatonin. If you're on the cancer journey, a lack of sleep can weaken the immune system that stands between your recovery and death.

Third, you must keep moving! Movement allows the lymphatic system to do its job removing the trash from your body. In fact, almost every system in your body is enhanced and strengthened through exercise. Unfortunately, the sedentary lifestyle is the new smoking, and it's a killer. For the cancer patient, movement is absolutely critical.

Fourth, your nutritional choices are among the most important decisions you will make each day. God has provided you the bounty of nature to nourish and build your immune system with phytochemicals, antioxidants, vitamins, minerals, proteins, and so much more. To feed on that bounty you must plan your meals around the idea that food is medicine. If you have a sweet tooth or a constant craving for carbs, you need to acquire the discipline of Daniel and exercise it daily. Remember, there are foods that feed cancer and foods that prevent cancer—learn and know the difference and make better choices. Unfortunately, the Standard American Diet (SAD) is cancer-promoting; SAD allows the witch to fly on her broom. Embrace the power of plants and make the dietary changes necessary for your body to heal at the cellular level.

Fifth, don't overlook the proper care of your mental and emotional well-being. Emotions impact your immune system in both positive and negative ways. If you're in conflict with someone, take steps to repair the relationship before the sun goes down on your anger. Even if you've deeply buried your emotional pain, your body is keeping score.

Keep in mind that there is always an emotional aspect to cancer, and emotional stress is the most underestimated risk factor that can suppress the body's immune system. Patients who are optimistic and utilize their faith to manage their emotions will improve their chances of recovery. In the cancer journey, one must put on the whole armor of God and wear it into battle. It takes strong faith and discipline to change one's lifestyle habits.

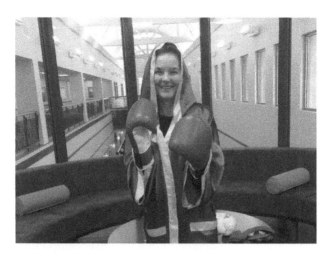

Beating cancer was the toughest battle of my life.

Turn to faith to help you with the emotional aspects of the journey. Even after surviving my cancer journey, I am not promised tomorrow. Neither are you. But if you are a child of God, you are promised something much better: eternal life. Cancer may indeed be a gift—the best thing that ever happened to you. Or it might be your ticket to heaven, that place over the rainbow where cancer is nonexistent. Either way, you win if you are in Christ.

Sixth, keep an attitude of gratitude. The power of thankfulness is a step you can't ignore. Remember to look for silver linings, even in the cancer journey. A spirit that remains hopeful, thankful, and joyful in the midst of the storm will survive and even thrive. Holocaust survivors have taught us that *hope* is a most powerful mindset.

Seventh, detoxify your body and home. Toxins exist in your food, your water, and your air. In fact, the most toxic substances you encounter might be found in your own home. If you want to help your immune system work efficiently, you must reduce your toxic load. If the human body is exposed to more toxins than its filtering systems can handle, diseases such as cancer may result. Be preventative by implementing daily and periodic detoxing.

Also, consider the potential impact of electromagnetic fields on your body and immune system. Turn off your Wi-Fi at night and follow the recommendations for responsible cell phone use. Don't fall into the trap of thinking EMFs are harmless because they're invisible. Use technology responsibly.

Eighth, rebuild and maintain a healthy gut. Eliminate those things in your life that weaken the gut lining and make wise nutritional choices to restore your microbiome. Remember that 70 percent of the immune system is located in the gut—the center of your health. If you've been through chemotherapy, you must proactively work to protect and restore your gut. Unfortunately, what happens in the gut doesn't stay in the gut; it affects the entire body. Your gut is the key to your recovery and restoring your body to vibrant health.

These eight steps work synergistically to build and maintain the immune system. Toxins, negative emotions, and stress suppress the immune system, while proper hydration, nutrition, exercise, sleep, faith, gratitude, and a healthy gut enhance and build the immune system. The side effects of implementing these steps are only positive. In a cancer journey with so many negative side effects, we need all the positive effects we can get!

Beating Genetics

Be encouraged that your genes do not dictate your future. Your genes only determine if you are vulnerable to certain diseases. According to Dr. Ben Lynch, "We all have dirty genes, but we can change or clean up our gene expression by targeting them with lifestyle changes."[1]

If you are one of the fortunate few who beat cancer without resorting to conventional treatments such as surgery, chemo, or radiation, then good for you! You didn't have to poison your body to destroy the disease. In my journey, I've met patients who've beat cancer with no chemotherapy or radiation, and I applaud them. If, however, you had to use chemotherapy and other toxic treatments, you *must* develop a plan to restore your body to health. Your due diligence is not over when the doctor pronounces the wicked witch dead; you're not home yet. You must address the root cause of your illness and remedy the situation that allowed the cancer to thrive. If you want to make it home safely, correct what went wrong and stick to a plan of restoration.

If you don't want to be disabled down the road, recognize that what you do today will have an impact on your aging years. Don't wait until you get sick to start making changes in your life. I certainly wish I had changed my lifestyle habits sooner. I can't go back, but I *can* make changes going forward. Be proactive *before* you discover a health problem.

All these warnings and calls for lifestyle changes need to be balanced with a humorous story I once heard a pastor preach on heaven. A husband and wife are walking the streets of gold in heaven, basking in God's glory, and the husband says to his wife, "Honey, if you hadn't made us eat all that healthy food, we could have gotten here sooner!"

There's a big difference between being ready for God to bring you home when it's time and trying to get there sooner! Your journey will be appreciably more pleasant and productive if you're making every effort to restore and maintain good health while shooting for the 120 years.

Life Expectancy Decreases while Disability Increases

According to the Centers for Disease Control, life expectancy in the U.S. has declined the past few years.[2] After decades of increasing numbers, why are we now witnessing this decline? Modern medicine has certainly contributed to our longevity, so could it be that our lifestyle choices are contributing to this recent decline?

Recent data indicates death rates due to cancer are on the decline; however, chronic illnesses are on the rise in our country.[3] According to the U.S. Census Bureau, nearly one in five Americans are now disabled.[4] Dr. Leigh Erin Connealy recently stated, "The US is the world leader in chronic diseases."[5] Some of these diseases have no doubt been caused by our lifestyles. Chronic illness and disability are not good for our country or its economy, and it's especially not beneficial for accomplishing the mission that was given to the body of Christ in Matthew 28:16–20.

It's All About the Immune System

It's important that contemporary men and women take steps to strengthen their immune systems to prevent cancer and many other diseases. The immune system is front and center. We all harbor potentially cancerous cells in our bodies.[6] If our immune system is healthy and functions as it's meant to, like an army ready for combat, it can detect and destroy foreign invaders.

It takes many variables to weaken a person's immune system and allow cancer to thrive. Unfortunately, there is an occasional disconnect between conventional medicine and integrative medicine, and we desperately need both in the battle against cancer.

The eight steps presented here are designed to strengthen the immune system. While this book focuses on the wicked witch of cancer, following and implementing these steps can also prevent Alzheimer's, diabetes, autoimmune disorders, and heart disease while contributing to longevity and health. A healthy human body is self-regulating and self-repairing. Cancer and other major diseases are signs that the immune system has shifted from defense-and-repair mode to becoming defense-dominant and repair-deficient.

Typically, it's not just one thing that causes cancer. In my case, I found several things that I needed to remedy. I've learned much on the Yellow Brick Road. My cancer motivated me to closely examine my lifestyle and assess where I needed to make improvements. We all need to examine our lifestyle choices.

Instead of traveling toward the Emerald City, we need to get back to Eden and rediscover the basics of life. Once I received my diagnosis, I was willing to do anything to get well. Facing the reality of death gave me the resolve to make necessary changes to my habits and start controlling what goes into my mouth.

Change takes time, and it requires discipline. Some changes will increase your budget, while others won't. It costs relatively little (compared to treating cancer) to drink more water, sleep better, exercise more, eat healthier, utilize your faith, thank God daily for your blessings, reduce your toxic load, and protect your gut.

Only you can decide which strategies to implement.

Don't just ask what your doctor can do to improve your health; ask what *you* can do to help your doctor improve your health. After all, no doctor and no treatment can guarantee you a 100 percent chance of success. Neither can I. And your doctor has no control over your lifestyle. I can promise that each change you make will improve your chances of preventing and surviving cancer and preventing its recurrence.

The Doctor Prescribes:

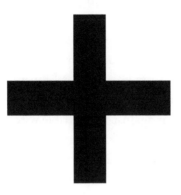

A Holistic Approach

We desperately need to use both the best of conventional medicine and well-researched integrative and holistic therapies in the fight against cancer. Recommendations from well-trained nutritionists and naturopathic doctors can be very valuable in the cancer journey. We must acknowledge that fighting cancer requires more than just surgery, radiation, and mixing chemicals. Enhancing the immune system to do its God-given job gives the patient more ammunition for the battle.

Dr. Robert L. Elliott

Return to Oz

Dorothy and I both had terrifying encounters with a tornado in our lives, and we both received lumps and bumps that took us on unexpected journeys. We met witches, lions, tigers, and bears (oh my) along the way. There were munchkins who cheered us on and sang for joy when the wicked witch died.

Dorothy realized that there was nothing in the Wizard's black bag that could send her home. Although I relied on many treatments from my doctors' black bags, I too learned that I must play a major role in my healing. Cancer patients must be their own best advocates and take action if they are to win the war against this terrible witch.

Dorothy had three faithful friends and Glinda to help her along the way. I also had those who helped me survive and thrive through the journey—my doctors, naturopaths, nutritionists, acupuncturists, and caring friends and family who faithfully prayed for me and supported me. My husband was my Tin Man who lifted my heart when mine was shattered.

Like the Scarecrow, I realized that I had a brain. So do you. The research is out there; you only have to find it. I used mine to connect the dots between nutrition, human anatomy and physiology, medical research, informed professional opinions, and the wisdom of God's Word. I feel that I've earned a degree from my journey—Doctor of Beating Cancerology from the School of Hard Knocks!

But like the Cowardly Lion, I needed the courage to follow through. My heavenly Lord—the Lion of Judah—gave me the nerve to face my treatments and the guidance to make it back home to safety.

The Wizard told Dorothy, "Don't pay attention to that man behind the curtain!" It turned out Oz the Great and Powerful was not a wizard at all. We must take the initiative to look behind the curtain and discover the causes of cancer and how to prevent and beat it. I had many Toto's who helped me pull back the curtain on cancer—medical researchers, scientists, nutritionists, doctors, and "The Truth About Cancer" series. Learning how the body works made a huge difference in my recovery.

Dorothy's journey was a nightmare she woke up from. Mine was real life. But we both learned many lessons along the Yellow Brick Road, with all its ups and downs, and steps forward and backward. I'm grateful for all I learned, but I don't want to travel this road again. And I hope and pray that I have helped you avoid this road by providing these eight steps as a road map.

Glinda told Dorothy, "You've always had the power to go back to Kansas." Her power was in her ruby-red slippers. Your power is in your God-given, self-healing, self-repairing body. Just as Dorothy clicked her heels together to activate the shoes' magic, by implementing these eight steps you allow your miraculous immune system to function as God intended.

Dorothy discovered that there's no place like home. I discovered that it's my job to take care of this amazing, self-healing home I've been given.

I know now that every day is a gift, and I don't want my time on earth to be cut short due to my own lack of discipline. My body is where I live, and it's my responsibility to take care of it. I'm striving for all 120 years of service that was granted to Moses. In the meantime, I am comforted, knowing that there is a place waiting for me over the rainbow.

"For I will restore health to you and heal you of your wounds," says the Lord.
Jeremiah 30:17

AFTERWORD

She Had to Find It Out for Herself

And lest I should be exalted above measure by the abundance of the revelations, a thorn in the flesh was given to me, a messenger of Satan to buffet me, lest I be exalted above measure. Concerning this thing I pleaded with the Lord three times that it might depart from me. And He said to me, "My grace is sufficient for you, for My strength is made perfect in weakness." Therefore most gladly I will rather boast in my infirmities, that the power of Christ may rest upon me.
—2 Corinthians 12:7–9

Moreover David said, "The LORD, who delivered me from the paw of the lion and from the paw of the bear, He will deliver me from the hand of this Philistine."
—1 Samuel 17:37

The simple believes everything, but the prudent gives thought to his steps.
—Proverbs 14:15 (esv)

With my first surgery around the corner, Alton felt that honesty was the best way to deal with his students at Clemson University. "I won't be here most of next week," he said to them, holding back tears. "It's not something that I planned, but my wife has been diagnosed with cancer. She's having surgery next week in Chicago." You could hear a pin drop in the classroom.

Frankly it was difficult for both of us to say the word "cancer."

At the end of class, many students came forward to offer my husband words of encouragement and prayer. Deshaun Watson, then Clemson's quarterback and soon-to-be Heisman nominee and NFL star, was the first to step forward. "AB, I'm so sorry about your wife," he said. "My mom had cancer a few years ago, and it was the hardest thing I've ever been through. She's better now. I'll be praying for your wife."

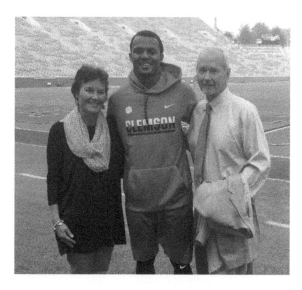

Former Clemson quarterback, Deshaun Watson, knows the sting of cancer.

"Why Didn't You Tell Her Before?"

Before my first surgery, I asked to meet with a chaplain at CTCA. When I stepped into the chaplain's office, I had a list of questions. I blurted them out in rapid succession, starting with my real concerns: Would all these treatments leave me disabled and negatively affect my quality of life?

I explained to him that the last fifteen years of my life had been centered on caring for my ailing parents and in-laws while holding a full-time job.

"I understand your fears of being disabled, with all you've been through," he responded. "Chemotherapy is a doable thing. Your medical records and bloodwork show that you are healthy. That will make a difference in your recovery."

"But if I'm so healthy, why did I get cancer?" I asked.

"Sometimes the *why* is hard to know, but I do know this: Patients who are healthy, have positive attitudes, and rely on their faith do much better than those who don't. If you're already overweight and suffering from diabetes, high blood pressure, and other problems, your body will have more problems with the chemo."

"Really? So, my good health habits that did not prevent my cancer will help me survive chemo?"

"Exactly. What other concerns do you have?"

"My husband—what will this do to him? We've been married almost forty years," I said, tears streaming down my face. "I'm not afraid of dying; I'm afraid of what this cancer will do to him."

"I understand," the chaplain said compassionately as he reached for my hand. "Anyone would be afraid. But that's where faith comes in. God will give both of you the strength to handle whatever comes your way."

I had to ask again. "How could a health nut like me end up with an aggressive and deadly cancer like this?"

"Ginny, consider it a gift from God. Sometimes God allows things in your life for you to help others. You have a platform as an author and speaker. Your experience in this journey can be a guiding light to others."

"But it's a gift I never wanted," I blurted. I remembered then I had said this twice before to Alton. The apostle Paul prayed three times for his thorn to be removed (2 Corinthians 12:7–8), and I was praying desperately this cancerous thorn would be taken from me. No one wants cancer. I wouldn't wish it on my worst enemy!

"Yes, I can see it now, your next book with this inscription—'It was the book I never wanted to write.'" He chuckled. "In time you will see the hand of God. I promise."

Near the end of *The Wizard of Oz*, when it appears that Dorothy has lost her only way home after the Wizard has sailed away helplessly in his hot air balloon, Glinda tells her that she's always had the power to go back to Kansas.

Indignant, the Scarecrow asks, "Then why didn't you tell her before?"

"Because she wouldn't have believed me. She had to learn it for herself," Glinda replies.

The Tin Man leans into his friend. "What have you learned, Dorothy?"

Dorothy thinks hard for a moment then gives a rather convoluted answer that is later summed up in the more memorable phrase "There's no place like home."

"But that's so easy," Scarecrow says. "I should have thought of it *for* you."

"I should have felt it in my heart," says the Tin Man.

"No," says Glinda, "she had to find it out for herself."

Some lessons cannot simply be taught in a classroom or in the Munchkins' town square; they must be learned in the crucible of life through intense, transformational experience.

I learned all that I've shared in these pages on my cancer journey. But the Yellow Brick Road is no Sunday stroll through the park; it's a terrifying, heart-in-your-throat roller coaster ride of physical and emotional ups and downs. This unexpected journey would require me to exercise my faith at its deepest levels while making many difficult choices under constant threat of death.

Yet I finally stepped out of the woods and into the sun with more knowledge, greater wisdom, and a stronger faith. Don't get me wrong—no one wants cancer. I pray you never have to travel this road (or travel it again) but can learn from "my bads."

My husband repeatedly tells me, "You're not the woman I married!" He's right. Thank God! But as Elisabeth Elliot, who lost her husband to martyrdom, wisely said, "The difference is Christ in me—not me in a different set of circumstances."

The Path of Blind Trust

In these few remaining pages, I want to share a bit more about my specific cancer journey in the hopes that it might benefit you should you ever find yourself on the Yellow Brick Road.

After an MRI was done to determine the extent of my cancer, I left work early one day to get the results from my surgeon.

"I'm afraid there is more than we expected," he said. "Your tumor has already planted another tumor. And your lymph nodes appear to be involved as well as your upper right torso."

I couldn't move. My mind went blank. All I could manage to say was, "I don't believe you. Show me the MRI."

The surgeon escorted me to an office and pulled up my MRI on a large screen. It was horrifying. The mass in question looked like a tornado on a TV weather map. Could that really be me? I had never danced with death before. *Wake up*, I told myself. *It's just a bad dream.*

I wandered out of the office and waited for what seemed like hours for Alton to pick me up. I was barely treading water, my head bobbing just above the surface as I gasped for air. When my husband arrived, I climbed into the cab of his red truck and stammered, "It's already spread—maybe to other parts of my body—my lungs, my organs."

We were running short on time to catch a plane to Chicago for a second opinion. Alton simply held my hand, and we both cried as he drove down I-85 to the airport in Atlanta. "It's hard for me to hear," he finally said, "but I know God will use it for good. . . . He's always been there for us."

I had been dropped into the middle of Oz, my head reeling as I set out on the Yellow Brick Road. At times the woods seemed to close in around me, dark and foreboding with no glimmer of light or hope. Sometimes the path grows darker before we see any light. Yet God expects us to trust Him even when we can't see His hand. That's always been tough for me; I prefer to see what's ahead. This road was populated by wild beasts that have been known to devour unsuspecting travelers. And little dogs, too.

This was a true path of blind trust. But having to trust in the midst of life's deepest struggles strengthens one's faith and causes shallow roots to grow. The tougher the trial, the deeper the roots of our faith must grow. As I walked this path, I began to see life in a whole new light, though the light was faint at first. I was basically walking blind, with no yellow bricks to guide my way.

Lions, Tigers, and Bears—Oh My!

Who's afraid of lions and tigers and bears? Frankly, I was. I tried to be brave going into my first surgery, but I feared the worst. The first words from my lips after waking from the anesthesia: "How many nodes were taken?"

"Just two, dear. Just two." I felt the warmth of Dr. Amin's hand. "We won't know until the lab results come back Wednesday, but they looked good. I was able to get both tumors. The lab results will let me know if I cleared the margins."

I had taken two steps forward along the road.

Two days later, she reported, "The results are back, and the lymph nodes are clear. We needed to clear the margins in nine areas. We cleared them in seven, but still have two to clear. When you return for surgery in ten days, I will begin in those two areas. If I cannot clear the margins then, a mastectomy must be done."

Three steps back.

Two days after the second surgery to clear the remaining margins and reconstruct my breasts, Dr. Amin called. "We cleared the margins," she said.

Two steps forward. Praise God from whom all blessings flow!

But surgery was a drop in the bucket compared to what was to come: chemotherapy, the roaring Lion of my journey. This was the one thing in life I never, ever wanted to experience. I had practiced healthy habits to prevent things like this, and yet here I sat, strapped in a chair like a prisoner on death row.

Many times, I hoped and prayed that this cup, this chemo, would pass from me. If my tumor was slow growing and nonaggressive, surgery and a few changes in lifestyle would have been my choice. Indeed, with every fiber of my being I wanted to get off this road and take the all-natural route. But my tumor was aggressive. I was forced to look the terrible Lion in the eye.

Before going ahead with the chemo, my husband and I prayed about it daily. Alton kept reminding me, "How many cancer patients do you know who are living today who used chemo?"

"Many," I said.

"How many people do you know with aggressive or metastatic cancer who've chosen the all-natural route who are alive today?"

"Not too many."

Let's be honest. Both ends of the spectrum have their share of casualties. Patients have died despite undergoing chemotherapy and radiation treatments, and patients have died because natural treatments couldn't bring the cancer under control before it spread throughout the body.

The Lion would soon devour my immune system; I could only pray that it also consumed the cancer. With recommended lifestyle changes and vitamin C infusions, I would have a fighting chance to survive the toxic clutches of the roaring beast.

I took an active part in the battle and researched everything I could do to help the chemo work while lessening the side effects.

Preparation for the Lion

Alton and I returned to Chicago for my first chemotherapy treatment. Colleen, my nutritionist, gave me lots of advice on foods to avoid during the course of chemo and afterward—mainly acidic-type foods. "We need for you to eat nutritious foods even if you don't feel like eating. And remember to hydrate with water before, during, and after each treatment."

I was also given supplements to take after chemo to help with the neuropathy in my hands and feet. Little did I know then that L-glutamine powder and L-carnitine capsules would be such lifesavers during my chemo regimen.

Then it was time to sign the consent papers. Oh my. These were the hardest papers I've ever signed. So many tough decisions, so many pages listing the possible side effects, including death. When would it all end?

I remembered an interview I did with Joni Eareckson Tada after her journey with breast cancer. I had asked, "What advice can you give someone who's about to receive chemotherapy?" Here's her response:

> Having a good frame of mind helps! It helps to remember that the "poisonous drugs" being infused into your body are actually there to kill and eradicate an even more dangerous enemy: cancer. Mark 16:18 is a curious verse

when you relate it to chemotherapy, for it says of those who trust God, "when they drink deadly poison, it will not hurt them at all." When you're in chemo, take a good inspirational book to read, plenty of healthy snacks, and a big bottle of fresh, cool water. And while you're in chemo, look for ways to pray for the other patients near you; get to know their names and encourage them. Any trial seems lighter when you shift focus off "it" and onto others.[1]

Good advice. I tried focusing my attention on a young mother who was fighting my same cancer. I shared encouraging words to lighten her load as she battled this enemy for her children. I also looked for others in my path whom I could encourage and lift in prayer, even those along the way who had no faith.

Chemotherapy, Round One

Alton and I began the next morning on our knees. "Protect Ginny as she takes the chemotherapy mixture," my husband pleaded. "May it not harm her body. May she not get sick. May she come out strong." We then walked a few miles that morning to help relieve anxiety. My goal was to walk a few miles before and after each treatment.

After an all-organic breakfast in CTCA's cafeteria, we headed to the infusion lab. My chemotherapy port—a small device that's implanted under the skin near the heart to allow easy access to the bloodstream—was ready to receive, but I was still struggling with uncertainties. Would the chemotherapy damage my brain? My lungs? My heart?

This felt like three steps backward.

After administering the pre-medications, my nurse suited up in protective gown, gloves, and cap. Then she grabbed the four bags labeled "TOXIC DANGER."

"Why are you suiting up?" I asked.

"If any of these substances were to leak, it would burn me."

"And you're going to infuse these toxic chemicals into a vein close to my heart?"

This was a real life-or-death situation. To try to treat the cancer with only natural substances meant possible death, but to submit to chemotherapy could also mean death—a real catch-22. It took every bit of faith I had to allow the nurse to begin those drips. I would later write this book in hopes that you never find yourself in similar circumstances.

"I've got an idea," I said to the nurse, smiling. "Why don't we switch places? I'll suit up with the HAZMAT gear, and you can sit here." Humor always helps!

We tried to keep in mind Jesus's words, "When they drink deadly poison, it will not hurt them at all." And just as that nurse was wearing her protective gear, I had put in place many protections as recommended by others: vitamin C infusion the day before, increased hydration, good nutrition, exercise, supplements, and the whole armor of God to go into battle.

My husband gently held my hand through the entire ordeal. I remember sensing the tears in his soul. Chemo was hard for me to do, but it was also hard for him to watch. Sometimes watching a loved one endure a trial is harder than being the one in the hot seat. I'm not sure whose role is tougher—the caregiver's or the patient's. My husband was a wonderful caregiver.

We shared moments of nerve-induced laughter that day and, with all that hydration, many trips to the restroom with my entourage of pole and tubes trailing behind me. After five premeds and four toxic brews had passed through my body, the eight-hour marathon was over. The procedure went better than we had hoped. Amazingly, I had shown no side effects during the treatment.

Though it was the longest day of my life, I had taken five steps forward.

Boosting Red Blood Cells

After a wonderful family trip to Kauai, where I was able to hike three miles in the Waimea Canyon, I returned to Chicago for my third chemo treatment. This time I was advised to add acupuncture to my schedule to boost my red blood cell count. My oncologist warned me that if my red blood cell count fell to the 5–7 range, I would need a blood transfusion. My doctor at home, Dr. Passini, prescribed for me compounded vitamin B-12 shots. Alton did not like being the one who administered them.

My white blood cells were fine after being given the Neulasta shot. This shot is the reason so many cancer patients quickly return to work. However, my red blood cells were barely hovering above ten. I needed to be proactive to avoid a blood transfusion, so I also added acupuncture at home. (Acupuncture is also helpful in minimizing neuropathy.) A few months after chemotherapy was finished, I stopped the acupuncture treatments and B-12 shots. On the next visit, my red blood cells dropped from 12 to 11. After seeing these results, I restarted both the acupuncture and B-12 shots, and my levels returned to 12. My situation is just one case study, but again, more research needs to be done regarding how acupuncture and B-12 shots can aid a patient during the cancer journey.

Get a Second Opinion for All Treatments

When I returned home after my fourth round of chemo, I scheduled an appointment with a local oncologist, Dr. Jeffrey Giguere, for a second opinion on my chemo. It's important to always seek a second opinion on any cancer diagnosis, surgery, and chemotherapy regimen.

Dr. Giguere was surprised I'd just come back from my fourth chemo and was able to lift my head off the pillow, walk three miles, and appear as though nothing had happened the day before. "Your chemo regimen is one of the toughest on the body," he said. "Most of my patients are begging me to stop after three or four rounds. So what are you doing differently?"

I explained about the vitamin C infusions, supplements, acupuncture, B-12 shots, water, exercise, etc.

"I'm not trained in that," he said. "But whatever you are doing, it's agreeing with you. I wouldn't advise you to stop. I do advise my patients to hydrate and exercise, because I know those two things make a difference."

"What is your opinion about the mixture of the four chemos I'm being given?" I asked.

"I would prescribe three of those, but not the fourth, Perjeta. New research has proven it has no value in your situation. Perjeta is best used when you have a tumor that needs to be shrunk before surgery."

I was really glad I'd made that appointment. Always get a second opinion on each important decision concerning your care. I wish I had done it sooner. Dr. Giguere's philosophy was my philosophy: no more chemo than necessary!

Remember, as the patient, you are always in charge. It's your body, and no one cares about it more than you. You must be your own best advocate. Oncologists are just like us—they all have their opinions. Get more than one opinion.

Two steps forward.

The Future of Cancer Treatments

I did not know about the benefits of using genomic testing to determine which chemotherapy agents will work best in targeting your cancer when first diagnosed, but I highly recommend paying out of pocket for this amazing test. Through a blood sample, a lab is able to separate your cancer cells and grow them in a petri dish. Then according to Dr. James Forsythe, the lab can determine the best chemotherapy drugs to target your cancer, the best targeted agents and immunotherapies that work with your cancer, and the supplements and hormone therapies that may help kill your cancer.[2]

Since most chemotherapies poison and weaken the immune system, you've only got one good shot at killing your cancer. Most insurance companies will only pay for this test if the first rounds of chemotherapy don't work. It would be in your best interest if insurance companies would pay for this test upfront and avoid patients being poisoned twice! But until then, be proactive. This test is well worth the cost.

Sixth-Round Kickback

After transferring my future treatment to the Atlanta offices of CTCA, my new oncologist said, "I looked over your records from Chicago, and I recommend a change. I feel the Perjeta is not needed."

This oncologist and I were on the same page. Two steps forward. I'd already removed it from the advice of Dr. Giguere.

He then ordered my final chemotherapy. My oncology nurse warned me that the sixth chemo could kick your tail. And he was right. Two steps back.

That night, I was terribly weak. I leaned over and whispered to Alton, "If I should die tonight, I just want you to know that you've been the best husband any woman could have." I honestly felt that I might take my last breath.

But in a few days, I was back to walking.

That's when the nerve endings in my feet began to let me know they were there. It's called neuropathy, and it's a bear. So, my new naturopathic doctor suggested I soak my feet three to four times a week in a half-and-half mixture of warm water and apple cider vinegar. And it worked!

Two steps forward.

An Unexpected Scare

I returned three weeks later to CTCA for an infusion of Herceptin and for tests related to a cough that had started after my second chemo. The pulmonary function test and chest x-ray indicated there were problems, so the pulmonary specialist asked me to stay a few extra days for additional tests.

Two steps back.

Oh, the fears that a cancer journey generates. Not once, but numerous times. I knew breast cancer can easily spread to the lungs.

When the results came back, the doctor said, "Asthma. You have adult-onset asthma. It may be chemo-induced."

"Praise God!" I shouted with a smile.

Two steps forward. Asthma never looked so good. And it was temporary.

My next visit to CTCA Atlanta revealed some amazing results concerning my bloodwork. Within six weeks after completing the final round of harsh chemo drugs, my red and white blood cells and platelets were all back within normal ranges. Dr. Kenna Barber called me her "rock star cancer patient"! Cancer patients given my chemo regimen generally require two to five years for their blood counts to return to normal.

Two steps forward—or so I thought.

Radiation: The Ferocious Tiger

It was now time to discuss radiation to my breast. My first oncologist had said, "If it's cancer, we've caught it early. After a lumpectomy and a little radiation, you'll be good to go." From that first mention of radiation, I assumed it would be targeting only the small area from where we had removed the tumor (a little radiation). So, I was shocked at what I learned next.

My new CTCA radiologist told me, "We will be radiating your entire breast from top to bottom and side to side—middle of your chest to under your arm—for thirty treatments."

This news put me between a rock and a hard place. I was not willing to do the radiation that extensively. I returned home distraught.

Four big steps back.

My Bible study group and two pastors laid hands on me and prayed that I would make the right decision and have peace about it. If I chose not to undergo the radiation, the cancer might return. If I went through with it, the radiation could cause secondary cancers and other issues. It felt like death if I do, death if I don't. Such dilemmas are the everyday life of most cancer patients.

A year earlier, my own mother had died from the radiation administered during her cancer treatment. Quite honestly, though, she would have died anyway.

Derryck McLuhan, who had lost his wife not to her cancer but to the side effects of the radiation, gave me another option to consider. He said that he knew of some women who were using frankincense diluted in coconut oil rubbed over the breast in place of radiation. If you Google "frankincense," you will see that research shows it can kill some nonaggressive cancer cells. An integrative practitioner in the Chicago area also suggested I add myrrh and sandalwood oil to the mixture, as some people respond more to one oil than another.

If frankincense and myrrh were good enough for the baby Jesus, I decided they were good enough for me. After doing my research, I decided to forgo the radiation.

Instead, I would apply the frankincense mixture nightly while rebuilding my immune system through lifestyle changes to help target any residual cancer. Since the chemo had already damaged my lungs, I sincerely wanted to avoid doing further damage with radiation. Quality of life was an important goal for me from the beginning.

I felt God had provided both my answer and the peace in my heart. And such is the journey of a cancer patient. There are many tough decisions to be made along the Yellow Brick Road, and each person must make his or her own choices after consulting with their doctor, doing their own research, and talking with God. I know many who've had minimal to no issues with radiation. In addition, the newer machines, which allow a woman to lie prone for radiation, offer more protection to the areas near a woman's breasts. This is a blessing for many.

Sometimes radiation is what saves a person's life. I met a woman who had an inoperable tumor that was unresponsive to chemo, so her radiologist used radiation to cut off the blood supply to the tumor and kill it. In my case, radiation was advised as a way of killing off any residual cancer cells, but it likely came with a host of negative side effects, some of which would affect my already damaged lungs. I was convinced that the risks for me far exceeded the benefits. But not doing it meant I must work harder to change my lifestyle.

Another sure way to avoid radiation is to remove the entire breast. Mastectomies have their advantages, as my radiologist reminded me. Breast cancer patients are told this up front. If you don't want radiation, choose the mastectomy option.

However, I elected to keep my breast, reject radiation, and work to help my immune system destroy any remaining cancer cells, and the Holy Spirit gave Alton and me peace about the decision. Our decision has been confirmed time and time again.

Final confirmation came when Dr. Kenna Barber spoke these words after hearing my final decision: "You have done everything we have asked you to do in fighting cancer, except the radiation. You have made your decision, now move on knowing that people like you are the ones who beat cancer. They research, they change their lifestyles, and they become their own best advocate. I'm proud of you, as you are one of my most conscientious patients."

Five bold steps forward.

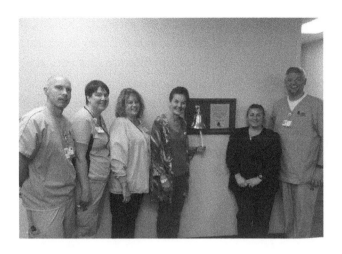

Thanks to these compassionate nurses who cheered me on.

Ding-Dong! The Witch Is Dead

There's nothing like ringing that bell off the wall. It's a traditional celebration for a cancer patient when one completes his or her treatments in the infusion lab. I'm not sure which was better, finishing that last bag of chemicals or the next week when they removed my port, my little buddy that had been lodged next to my heart. That port was a blessing and a necessity, but I was overjoyed to unfriend it and be a normal human again. I actually sang "Victory in Jesus" all the way down to the surgery room to have it removed.

Five steps forward.

The best news came after a post-chemotherapy MRI of my breasts. Dr. Panicker exclaimed, "You are cancer free." It was as if he had said, "You can live again."

Ten steps forward!

"Cancer free" means they can't detect any observable cancer, but I would be closely watched for some time. With an aggressive cancer like mine had been, I was warned this witch could return with a vengeance. This is why lifestyle changes were so important to me. New, healthier habits were my best chance of survival. I would go back as much as possible to the Garden of Eden.

The Snarling Bear of my journey, the estrogen-blocking pill and its side effects, would extend my journey on the Yellow Brick Road another five years. Five more years of three steps forward and two steps back, but the 40 percent reduction in recurrence made it worth it.

But the undeniable truth was that I had stood toe to toe with a formidable foe and won. With God at my side, and the help of both conventional and integrative medicine, we had slain the Wicked Witch. At least for now.

Praise God, from whom all blessings flow!
Thomas Ken, "Glory to Thee, My God, This Night"

NOTES

Chapter 1: Risk Factors: What about This Baptist Lifestyle?

1   Sarah Bosley, "Worldwide Cancer Cases Expected to Soar by 70% over Next 20 Years," *The Guardian*, February 3, 2014, www.theguardian.com/society/2014/feb/03/worldwide-cancer-cases-soar-next-20-years (accessed January 11, 2019).

2   Patrick Quillin, "Beating Cancer with Nutrition" keynote address at The Truth About Cancer Live, Orlando, Florida, October 5–7, 2017.

3   Honor Whiteman, "1 in 2 People Will Develop Cancer in Their Lifetime," *Medical News Today*, February 4, 2015, www.medicalnewstoday.com/articles/288916.php_(accessed January 14, 2019.)

4   "Breast Cancer Risk and Prevention," *American Cancer Society*, www.cancer.org/cancer/breastcancer/detailedguide/breast-cancer-risk-factors (accessed January 14, 2019.)

5   Preetha Anand et al, "Cancer Is a Preventable Disease that Requires Major Lifestyle Changes," *Pharmaceutical Research* 25, no. 9 (September 2008): 2097–2116.

Chapter 2: Hydrating Your Body

1   Yair Bar David, Benjamin Gesundheit, Jacob Urkin et al, "Water Intake and Cancer Prevention," *Journal of Clinical Oncology*, no. 2 (January 15, 2004): 383–385.

2   Reiping Tang et al, "Physical Activity, Water Intake and Risk of Colorectal Cancer in Taiwan: A Hospital-Based Case-Control Study," *International Journal of Cancer* 82, no. 4 (August 12, 1999): 484–489.

3   Dominique Michaud et al, "Fluid Intake and Risk of Bladder Cancer in Men," *New England Journal of Medicine* 340, no. 18 (May 6, 1999): 1390–1397.

4   "ACS Guidelines on Nutrition and Physical Activity for Cancer Prevention," *American Cancer Society*, www.cancer.org/healthy/eat-healthy-get-active/

acs-guidelines-nutrition-physical-activity-cancer-prevention.html (accessed January 2014).

5   Susan Kleiner, "Water: An Essential but Overlooked Nutrient," *Journal of Nutrition and Dietetics* 99, no. 2 (February 1999): 200–06.

6   Ocean Robbins, "The Truth About Drinking Water and What You Need to Know to Be Safe," *The Food Revolution Blog*, November 22, 2016, https://foodrevolution.org/blog/taking-action/truth-about-drinking-water (accessed January 24, 2019).

7   Tony Robbins interview, *The Water Cure*, http://www.watercure.com/media/interview.html (accessed April 6, 2019).

8   Ibid.

9   Fereydoon Batmanghelidj, *Your Body's Many Cries for Water* (Falls Church: Global Health Solutions, 2008), 182.

10 Ibid.

11 "Noble Prize Winner, Dr. Otto Warburg: On the Cause of Cancer," *Apex Health,* August 22, 2017. https://apexhealth.life/nobel-prize-winner-dr-otto-warburg-on-the-cause-of-cancer/ (accessed January 14, 2019).

12 Nancy Hearn, "Body Oxygenation for Health and Vitality—4 How To's," *Water Benefits Health*, www.waterbenefitshealth.com/body-oxygenation.html (accessed January 14, 2019).

13 Rachel Arthur, "'Bottled Water Is America's Favorite Drink!' Bottled Water Takes Top Spot in US," Beveragedaily.com, June 1, 2018, www.beveragedaily.com/Article/2018/06/01/Bottled-water-takes-top-spot-in-US-in-2017 (accessed January 14, 2019).

14 Don Colbert, *The Seven Pillars of Health* (Lake Mary: Siloam, 2007), 33.

15 Batmanghelidj, *Your Body's Many Cries,* 108.

16 Ibid., 139.

17 Ty M. Bollinger, *The Truth About Cancer: What You Need to Know about Cancer's History, Treatment, and Prevention* (Carlsbad, CA: Hay House, 2016).

18 Igor Smirnov, "MRET Activated Water and its Successful Application for Prevention Treatment and Enhanced Tumor Resistance in Oncology," *European Journal of Scientific Research* 16, no. 4 (2007): 575–583.

19 Gina Bria interview with Jonathan Landsman, "Dehydration—The Truth About Drinking Water and Avoiding Disease," *Natural Health 365*, April 23, 2018, www.naturalhealth365.com/dehydration-disease-2537.html (accessed January 14, 2019).

20 Ibid.

21 Diana Price, "Hydrate for Good Health," *Cancer Fighters Thrive*, www.cancerfightersthrive.com/hydrate-for-good-health (accessed January 14, 2019).

Chapter 3: Restoring and Rebuilding Your Body with Deep Sleep

1   Daniel Amen and Tana Amen, "Gratitude and Brain Fit," *YouTube*, December 11, 2016, www.youtube.com/watch?v=XiSCkiq7gGs (accessed January 14, 2019).

2   Interview with Prof. Russell Foster, *University of Oxford*, www.ox.ac.uk/research/research-in-conversation/healthy-body-healthy-mind/russell-foster (accessed January 14, 2019).

3   Colbert, *The Seven Pillars of Health*, 38–39.

4   Dr. Russell Foster, "Why Do We Need Sleep?" speech at doTERRA Convention in Salt Lake City, September 15, 2016.

5   Ibid.

6   Michael Breus, "Sleep Problems May Contribute to Cognitive Decline," *The Sleep Doctor*, August 11, 2012, www.thesleepdoctor.com/2012/08/11/sleep-problems-may-contribute-to-cognitive-decline (accessed January 14, 2019).

7   Yasmin Anwar, "Everything You Need to Know about Sleep, but Are Too Tired to Ask," *Berkeley News*, October 17, 2017, http://news.berkeley.edu/2017/10/17/whywesleep (accessed January 14, 2019).

8   "Could Getting a Good Night's Sleep Reduce Your Risk of Cancer," *Registry Partners*, April 27, 2018, www.registrypartners.com/could-getting-a-good-nights-sleep-reduce-your-risk-of-cancer (accessed January 14, 2019).

9   Thomas Erren et al, "Shift Work and Cancer: The Evidence and the Challenge," *Deutsches Arzteblatt International* 107, no. 38 (September 2010): 657–662.

10 "Rotating night shift work can be hazardous to your health," *Science Daily*, January 5, 2015, www.sciencedaily.com/releases/2015/01/150105081757.htm (accessed January 1, 2019).

11 Michael Breus interview with Peggy Sarlin, "The Wakeful Brain: How Sleep Affects Memory and Cognition," *Awakening from Alzheimer's*, September 30, 2017.

12 Ibid.

13 Alan Christianson, "Adrenal 101: The Myths and the Science Behind Adrenal Stress and Fatigue," *Dr. Christianson.com*, http://drchristianson.com/adrenal-101-the-myths-and-the-science-behind-adrenal-stress-fatigue (accessed January 14, 2019).

14 Ibid.

15 Chris Wark, "Sleep with Me: How Much Sleep Do You Really Need?" *Chris Beat Cancer*, www.chrisbeatcancer.com/sleep-with-me (accessed April 5, 2019).

16 Michigan State University, "Melatonin Boost a Key to Fighting Breast Cancer," *Science Daily*, August 23, 2016, www.sciencedaily.com/releases/2016/08/160823125354.htm (accessed January 14, 2019).

17 Bo Christensen, "Melatonin Could Be Overlooked Treatment for Cancer," *Science Nordic,* June 1, 2015, http://sciencenordic.com/melatonin-could-be-overlooked-treatment-cancer (accessed January 14, 2019).

18 Michael Breus, "The Latest on Blue Light and Sleep," *The Sleep Doctor*, November 6, 2017, www.thesleepdoctor.com/2017/11/06/latest-blue-light-sleep (accessed January 14, 2019).

19 Katie Ressler, "Why Should Sleep Be a Priority for Cancer Patients," *Cancer Fighters Thrive*, March 2018, www.cancerfightersthrive.com/sleep-priority-cancer-patients/#tips?utm_source=March+2018 (accessed January 14, 2019).

20 "The Truth About Alcohol and Sleep," The Sleep Doctor, November 15, 2017, https://thesleepdoctor.com/2017/11/15/truth-alcohol-sleep (accessed April 8, 2019).

Chapter 4: Moving Your Body toward Optimum Health

1 Leigh Erin Connealy, *The Cancer Revolution: A Groundbreaking Program to Reverse and Prevent Cancer* (Boston: Da Capo Press, 2017), 115–119.

2 Ibid., 118.

3 Samantha Brooks et al, "Late-life Obesity Is Associated with Smaller Global and Regional Gray Matter Volumes: A Voxel-Based Morphometric Study," *International Journal of Obesity* 37 (2013): 230–236.

4 Robert Pendergrast, *Breast Cancer: Reduce Your Risk with Foods You Love* (North Augusta: Penstokes Press, 2010), 27.

5 Ibid.

6 Ibid., 29–30.

7 Ibid., 30.

8 Joseph Maroon, "The Brain and Exercising," *Dr. Maroon*, www.josephmaroon.com/the-brain-exercising (accessed January 19, 2019).

9 "Diet and Physical Activity: What's the Cancer Connection?" American Cancer Society, www.cancer.org/cancer/cancer-causes/diet-physical-activity/diet-and-physical-activity.html (accessed January 14, 2019).

10 Edward Laskowski, "How Much Should the Average Adult Exercise Every Day?" *Mayo Clinic Online*, www.mayoclinic.org/healthy-lifestyle/fitness/expert-answers/exercise/faq-20057916 (accessed January 14, 2019)

11 Chris Wark, chrisbeatcancer.com.

12 Robert Lustig interviewed by Dr. Joe Mercola, "Research Proves Causation—Sugar Consumption Increases Risk for Chronic Disease," *Mercola*, January 25, 2015, https://articles.mercola.com/sites/articles/archive/2015/01/25/sugar-increases-chronic-disease-risk.aspx (accessed January 14, 2019).

13 Clinical Oncology Society of Australia, "COSA Position Statement on Exercise and Cancer Care," May 2018, www.cosa.org.au/media/332488/cosa-position-statement-v4-web-final.pdf (accessed January 14, 2019).

14 Katie Dangerfield, "Exercise is 'Best Medicine' and Should Be Prescribed to Every Cancer Patient," *Global News*, May 27, 2018, https://globalnews.ca/news/4191157/cancer-exercise-best-medicine-researchers-australia (accessed January 14, 2019).

15 Robb Wolfe interviewed by Jason Prall, "The Human Longevity Project Documentary Series," May 11, 2018, https://humanlongevityfilm.com.

16 Datis Kharrazian interviewed by Jason Prall, "The Human Longevity Project Documentary Series," May 11, 2018, https://humanlongevityfilm.com.

17 Connealy, *The Cancer Revolution*, 302.

18 Loren Fishman and Ellen Saltonstall, *Yoga for Osteoporosis* (New York: W. W. Norton & Company, 2010), 27.

19 Ibid., 28.

20 Loren Fishman, *Healing Yoga: Proven Postures to Treat Common Ailments from Backache to Bone Loss, Shoulder Pain to Bunions, and More* (New York: W. W. Norton & Company, 2015).

21 Julia Buckley, "5 Healing Yoga Moves for Arthritis," *Community Table*, May 6, 2014, https://communitytable.parade.com/286249/juliabuckley/5-healing-yoga-moves-for-arthritis/ (accessed January 14, 2019).

22 Eva Norlyk Smith, "Yoga for Osteoporosis," *Yoga U Online,* www.yogauonline.com/yogau-wellness-blog/yoga-for-osteoporosis-interview-loren-fishman-md-and-ellen-saltonstall (accessed January 14, 2019).

23 Matt Riemann interviewed by Jason Prall, "The Human Longevity Project Documentary Series," May 11, 2018, https://humanlongevityfilm.com.

Chapter 5: Food as Powerful Medicine

1 Dr. Vincent Fortanasce, *The Anti-Alzheimer's Prescription* (New York: Gotham Books, 2008), 9.

2 Ibid., 37.

3 U.S. Department of Health and Human Services and U.S. Department of Agriculture, "Dietary Guidelines for Americans 2015–2020," *The Office of Disease Prevention and Health Promotion*, December 2015, https://health.gov/dietaryguidelines/2015/guidelines/chapter-1 (accessed January 15, 2019).

4 U. S. Department of Agriculture, "Choose My Plate," www.choosemyplate.gov/ (accessed January 14, 2019).

5   Betsy McKay and Suzanne Vranica, "Government Ads Urge Americans to Shed Pounds," *The Wall Street Journal*, March 10, 2004, www.wsj.com/articles/SB107888495735051075 (accessed April 5, 2019).

6   Dr. Ben Lynch, *Dirty Genes: A Breakthrough Program to Treat the Root of Your Illness and Optimize Your Health* (San Francisco: Harper One, 2018).

7   Colbert, *The Seven Pillars of Health*, 65.

8   "It's Easy to Add Fruits and Vegetables to Your Diet," *American Cancer Society*, www.cancer.org/healthy/eat-healthy-get-active/eat-healthy/add-fruits-and-veggies-to-your-diet.html (accessed January 14, 2019).

9   Harri Vainio and Elisabette Weiderpass, "Fruit and Vegetables in Cancer Prevention," *Journal of Nutrition and Cancer* 54, no. 1 (2006): 111–142; Gladys Block, Blossom Patterson, and Amy Subar, "Fruits, Vegetables, and Cancer Prevention: A Review of the Epidemiological Evidence," *Journal of Nutrition and Cancer* 18, no. 1 (1992): 1–29.

10   Cheryl Rock, Wendy Demark-Wahnefried, "Can Lifestyle Modification Increase Survival in Women Diagnosed with Breast Cancer?" *The Journal of Nutrition* 132, no. 11 (November 2002): 3504S–3509S; Jennifer Ligibel, "Lifestyle Factors in Cancer Survivorship," *Journal of Clinical Oncology* 30, no. 30 (October 20, 2012): 3697–3704.

11   William Li, "Can We Eat to Starve Cancer," *Ted Talks*, 2010, www.ted.com/talks/william_li/up-next (accessed January 14, 2019).

12   Ibid.

13   William Li, *Eat to Beat Disease* (New York: Grand Central Publishing, 2019), xxi.

14   Steven Jackson and Keith Singletary, "Sulforaphane Inhibits Human MCF-7 Mammary Cancer Cell Mitotic Progression and Tubulin Polymerization," *Journal of Nutrition* 134, no. 9 (September 2004): 2229–2236.

15   Zheng Dong, "Effects of Food Factors on Signal Transduction Pathways," *Biofactors* 12, nos. 1-4 (2000): 17–28.

16   Don Colbert, *Toxic Relief* (Lake Mary: Charisma House, 2012), 68.

17   American Cancer Society, *Nutrition and Prevention*, (New York: American Cancer Society, 1984).

18   Veronique Desaulniers, Heal Breast Cancer Naturally: Seven Essential Steps to Beating Breast Cancer (Indianapolis: TKC Publishing, 2014), 48.

19   Ibid., 48–49.

20   Jillian Levy, "4 Steps to Achieve Proper pH Balance," *Dr. Axe*, November 8, 2017, https://draxe.com/balancing-act-why-ph-is-crucial-to-health (accessed January 15, 2019).

21   Ann Kulze, "Beans—A Food to Revere," *Dr. Ann*, August 9, 2009, http://drannwellness.com/beans-a-food-to-revere/ (accessed January 2015, 2019).

22   Dan Buettner, *The Blue Zones: Lessons for Living Longer from the People Who've Lived the Longest* (Des Moines: National Geographic Society, 2008), 98.

23   Patrick Quillin, *Beating Cancer with Nutrition* (Carlsbad: Nutrition Times Press, revised 2005), 9.

24   Ibid.

25   Ibid., 85.

26   Ann Kulze, "Learn Why Chocolate Is So Amazing for You," *YouTube*, July 20, 2017, www.youtube.com/watch?v=XzOXmj-3Ilc&feature=youtu.be (accessed January 15, 2019).

Chapter 6: Fats, Gluten, Dairy, and Sugar

1   Mayo Clinic Staff, "Dietary Fats: Know Which Types to Choose," *Mayo Clinic*, February 2, 2018, www.mayoclinic.org/healthy-lifestyle/nutrition-and-healthy-eating/in-depth/fat/art-20045550 (accessed January 15, 2019).

2   Artemis Simopoulos, "The Importance of the Ratio of Omega-6/Omega-3 Essential Fatty Acids," *Biomedicine & Pharmacotherapy* 56, no. 8 (October 2002), 365–379.

3   Jillian Levy, "How to Balance Omega 3 6 9 Fatty Acids," *Dr. Axe*, January 27, 2019, https://draxe.com/how-to-balance-omega-3-6-9-fatty-acids (accessed October 25, 2019).

4   David Rose, Jodie Rayburn, Mary Ann Hatala, and Jeanne M. Connolly, "Effects of Dietary Fish Oil on Fatty Acids and Eicosanoids in Metastasizing Human Breast Cancer Cells," *Nutrition and Cancer* 22, no.2 (June 2, 1994), 131–141.

5   Joe Mercola, "Coconut Oil: This Cooking Oil Is a Powerful Virus-Destroyer and Antibiotic," *Mercola*, October 22, 2010, http://articles.mercola.com/sites/articles/archive/2010/10/22/coconut-oil-and-saturated-fats-can-make-you-healthy.aspx (accessed January 15, 2019).

6   Ian Prior, F. Davidson, C. E. Salmond Z. Czochanska, "Cholesterol, Coconuts, and Diet on Polynesian Atolls: A Natural Experiment: The Pukapuka and Tokelua Island Studies," *The American Journal of Nutrition* 34, no. 8 (August 1, 1981): 1552–1561.

7   Joshua Axe, "Coconut Oil Benefits for Your Brain, Heart, Joints and More!" *Dr. Axe*, May 21, 2018, https://draxe.com/coconut-oil-benefits (accessed January 15, 2019).

8   Kim Sooi Law et al, "The Effects of Virgin Coconut Oil as Supplementation on Quality of Life Among Breast Cancer Patients," *Lipids in Health and Disease* 13, no. 139 (August 27, 2014): 1–7.

9   Michael Donaldson, "Nutrition and Cancer: A Review of the Evidence for an Anti-Cancer Diet," *Nutrition Journal* 3, no. 19 (October 29, 2004).

10 U.S. Department of Health and Human Services and U.S. Department of Agriculture, "Dietary Guidelines for Americans 2015–2020."

11 Jillian Levy, "Gluten Intolerance Symptoms and Treatment Methods," *Dr. Axe*, July 10, 2018, https://draxe.com/whats-the-deal-with-gluten (accessed January 15, 2019).

12 Artemis Simopoulos, "The Importance of the Omega-6/Omega-3 Fatty Acid Ratio in Cardiovascular Disease and Other Chronic Diseases," *Experimental Biological Medicine* 233, no. 6 (June 1, 208): 674–688; Michel de Lorgeril and Patricia Salen, "New Insights into the Health Effects of Dietary Saturated and Omega-6 and Omega-3 Polyunsaturated Fatty Acids," *BMC Medicine* 10, no. 50 (May 21, 2012).

13 Robert Locke, "4 Health Reasons For Why American Milk is Banned in Europe," *Lifehack.org*, August 2, 2018; Haider Rizvi, "Cancer Link to rBGH Milk, Study Says," *Albion Monitor*, March 30, 1996.

14 Pendergrast, *Breast Cancer*, 21.

15 Rachel Johnson et al, "Dietary Sugars Intake and Cardiovascular Health: A Scientific Statement from the American Heart Association," circulation 120, no. 11 (September 15, 2009): 1011–1020.

16 David Jockers, "Fighting Cancer with Nutritional Ketosis," *The Truth About Cancer* in Anaheim, California, October 11, 2019.

17 Connecticut College, "Are Oreos Addictive? Research Says Yes," *Science Daily*, October 15, 2013, www.sciencedaily.com/releases/2013/10/131015123341.htm (accessed April 5, 2013).

18 Kelly Turner, *Radical Remission: Surviving Cancer Against All Odds* (New York: HarperCollins, 2014), 15.

19 Colleen Gill, "Sugar and Cancer," *Oncology Nutrition*, July 2014, www.oncologynutrition.org/erfc/healthy-nutrition-now/sugar-and-cancer (accessed January 15, 2019); Veronique DeSaulniers, "Cancer Cells Love Sugar 44 Times More Than Healthy Cells," *Breast Cancer Conqueror*, April 8, 2003, https://breastcancerconqueror.com/cancer-cells-love-sugar-44-times-more-than-healthy-cells (accessed January 15, 2019).

20 "Glucose Deprivation Activates Feedback Loop that Kills Cancer Cells, Study Shows," *Science Daily* (June 2016), www.sciencedaily.com/releases/2012/06/120626131854.htm (accessed January 15, 2019).

21 Murray Susser, "Cancer Cover-up? The Low Dose Chemotherapy Your Oncologist Isn't Telling You About," *The Truth About Cancer*, September 7, 2015, https://thetruthaboutcancer.com/low-dose-chemotherapy-alternative.

22 U.S. Department of Health and Human Services and U.S. Department of Agriculture, "Dietary Guidelines for Americans 2015–2020."

Chapter 7: Organics, Herbs, Oils, and Supplements

1   Kelly Adams, W. Scott Butsch, and Martin Kohlmeier, "The State of Nutrition at U.S. Medical Schools," *Journal of Biomedical Education*, vol. 2015 (January 11, 2015).

2   Russell Blaylock, "GMO Food—It's Worse Than We Thought," *YouTube*, December 23,2013, www.youtube.com/watch?v=wA2GhOCtmBE (accessed January 16, 2019).

3   Jonathan Amos, "French GM-Fed Rat Study Triggers Furore," BBC News, September 12, 2012, www.bbc.com/news/science-environment-19654825 (accessed January 16, 2019).

4   Joshua Axe, "Is Organic Really Better?" *Dr. Axe*, July 16, 2017, https://draxe.com/is-organic-really-better (accessed January 16, 2019).

5   Pendergrast, *Breast Cancer*, 72.

6   Ibid., 74–75.

7   Bruno Challier, J. M. Perarnau, J. F. Viel, "Garlic, Onion, and Cereal Fibre as Protective Factors for Breast Cancer," *European Journal of Epidemiology* 14, no. 8 (December 1998): 737–747.

8   Rebekah Edwards, "Spirulina Benefits: 10+ Reasons to Use This Superfood," *Dr. Axe*, June 25, 2018, https://draxe.com/spirulina-benefits (accessed January 16, 2019).

9   Robert Tisserand, "Frankincense Essential Oil and Cancer: Why EOs and Chemotherapy Don't Always Mix," *Robert Tisserand*, March 26, 2015, http://roberttisserand.com/2015/03/frankincense-essential-oil-and-cancer (accessed January 16, 2019).

10 Song Yao et al, "Association of Serum Level of Vitamin D at Diagnosis With Breast Cancer Survival," *JAMA Oncology* 3, no. 3 (August 8, 2016): 351–357.

11 Fishman and Saltonstall, *Yoga for Osteoporosis*, 39.

12 David Brownstein, *Iodine: Why You Need It* (W. Bloomfield: Medical Alternatives Press, 2014), 25.

13 David Jockers, "5 Ways Fermented Foods Reduce Risk of Cancer," *The Truth About Cancer*, May 28, 2018, https://thetruthaboutcancer.com/fermented-foods-reduce-cancer-risk (accessed January 16, 2019).

14 Michelle Martínez-Montemayor et al, "Ganoderma Lucidum (Reishi) Inhibits Cancer Cell Growth and Expression of Key Molecules in Inflammatory Breast Cancer, *Nutrition and Cancer* 63, no. 7 (September 2, 2011): 1085–1094.

15 Gary Deng et al, "A Phase I/II Trial of a Polysaccharide Extract from *Grifola frondosa* (Maitake mushroom) in Breast Cancer Patients: Immunological Effects," *Journal of Cancer Research and Clinical Oncology* 135, no. 9 (September 2009): 1215–1221.

16 David Jockers, "Are You Eating These 8 Nutrients That Block Cancer Metastasis?" *The Truth About Cancer*, February 16, 2017, https://thetruthaboutcancer.com/nutrients-block-cancer-metastasis/ (accessed January 16, 2019).

17 Ibid.

Chapter 8: Living Your Faith to Manage Stress and Emotions

1 Archibald Hart, "*The Hidden Link Between Adrenaline and Stress* (Nashville: Thomas Nelson, 1995), 3.

2 Ibid., 8.

3 Ibid., 9.

4 Razi Ann Berry interview with Brian Mowll, "How Emotional Hormones Play a Role in Diabetes," The Diabetes Summit, April 23–30, 2018.

5 Niki Gratix, *The 7 Steps to Healing Childhood Emotional Trauma and Building Resilience*, e-book (2015).

6 Vincent Felitti et al, "Relationship of Childhood Abuse and Household Dysfunction to Many of the Leading Causes of Death in Adults," *American Journal of Preventative Medicine* 14, no. 4 (May 1998): 245–258.

7 Ibid.

8 Dick Woodward, *30 Biblical Reasons Why God's People Suffer* (Hampton, VA: International Cooperating Ministries, December 2004), 18.

9 David Jeremiah, "31 Happiness Affirmations," DavidJeremiah.org, www.davidjeremiah.org/site/happiness/31-happiness-affirmations (accessed January 16, 2019).

10 Earl Nightingale, *The Essence of Success*, quoted in "The Fog of Worry," *Nightingale Conant,* www.nightingale.com/articles/the-fog-of-worry-only-8-of-worries-are-worth-it (accessed January 16, 2019).

11 Laura Harris Smith, *The 30-Day Faith Detox* (Minneapolis: Chosen, 2016), 17.

Chapter 9: God's Remedies for Healing Emotions

1 Joe Carter, "9 Things You Should Know About Prayer in the Bible," *The Gospel Coalition*, www.thegospelcoalition.org/article/9-things-you-should-know-about-prayer-in-the-bible (accessed March 12, 2019).

2 Daniel Amen, "This Is Your Brain on Meditation," *The Brain Warriors Way Podcast*, October 11, 2018, http://brainwarriorswaypodcast.com/this-is-your-brain-on-meditation (accessed January 16, 2019).

3   Lee Berk, D. L. Felten, S. A. Tan, B. B. Bittman, and J. Westengard, "Modulation of Neuroimmune Parameters During the Eustress of Humor-Associated Mirthful Laughter," *Alternative Therapeutic Health Medicine* 7, no. 2 (March 2001): 62–76.

4   Tor Rodriguez, "Laugh Lots, Live Longer," *Scientific American*, September 1, 2016, www.scientificamerican.com/article/laugh-lots-live-longer (accessed January16, 2019).

5   Mike Adams, "Laughter Is Good Medicine for Reducing Stress, Enhancing Brain Chemistry," *Natural News*, April 28, 2015, www.naturalnews.com/007551.html (accessed January 16, 2019).

6   "Laughter Therapy," *Cancer Treatment Centers of America*, www.cancercenter.com/treatments/laughter-therapy (accessed January 16, 2019).

7   Daisy Fancourt, Aaron Williamon, Livia A. Carvalho, Andrew Steptoe, Rosie Dow, and Ian Lewis, "Singing Modulates Mood, Stress, Cortisol, Cytokine and Neuropeptide Activity in Cancer Patients and Carers," *ECancer Medical Science*, December 18, 2015, https://doi.org/10.3332/ecancer.2016.631 (accessed January 16, 2019).

8   Rong Fang, Shengxuan Ye, Jiangtao Huangfu, and David P. Calimag, "Music Therapy Is a Potential Intervention for Cognition of Alzheimer's Disease," *National Center for Biotechnology Information*, www.ncbi.nlm.nih.gov/pmc/articles/PMC5267457 (accessed March 13, 2019).

9   Ali Le Vere, "How Music Can Support Brain Regeneration & Healing," *Green Med Info*, www.greenmedinfo.com/blog/how-music-can-support-brain-regeneration-healing (accessed March 13, 2019).

10 "Adverse Childhood Experience (ACE) Questionnaire," *The Anna Institute*, October 24, 2006, www.theannainstitute.org/Finding%20Your%20ACE%20Score.pdf (accessed January 16, 2019).

Chapter 10: Practicing Gratitude as an Attitude

1   Daniel Amen, "7 Ways to Remain Grateful All Year Long," *Amen Clinics*, November 17, 2017, http://www.amenclinics.com/blog/write-yourself-happy (accessed January 16, 2019).

2   Daniel Amen, "Using Gratitude to Change Your Brain," *The Daniel Plan*, November 20, 2017, http://danielplan.com/blogs/dp/using-gratitude-to-change-your-brain-2 (accessed January 16, 2019).

3   Douglas Main, "5 Scientifically Proven Benefits of Gratitude," *Newsweek*, November 25, 2015, www.newsweek.com/5-scientifically-proven-benefits-gratitude-398582 (accessed January 16, 2019).

4   "Gratitude Is Good Medicine," *UC Davis Health*, November 11, 2015, www.ucdmc.ucdavis.edu/medicalcenter/features/2015-2016/11/20151125_gratitude.html (accessed January 16, 2019).

5   Mikaela Conley, "Thankfulness Linked to Positive Changes in Brain and Body," ABC News, November 23, 2011, http://abcnews.go.com/Health/science-thankfulness/story?id=15008148 (accessed January 16, 2019).

6   Ibid.

7   Ibid.

8   William Shakespeare, *Othello*, act 3, scene 3.

9   Ann Voskamp, "Known by Our Gratitude," *YouTube*, November 23, 2014, www.youtube.com/watch?v=WTSHtEpMrto (accessed January 16, 2019).

Chapter 11: Reducing Environmental Toxins

1   Francis A. Schaeffer and Udo W. Middlemann, *Pollution and the Death of Man* (Wheaton: Tyndale House, 1970), 72.

2   John Calvin, commentary on Genesis 2:15 in *Commentaries on the First Book of Moses called Genesis* (Grand Rapids MI, 1948).

3   Billy Graham, "Does God Care About the Environment?" *Billy Graham Evangelistic Association*, https://billygraham.org/answer/does-god-care-about-the-environment (accessed January 16, 2019).

4   Dr. Joseph Pizzorno interviewed by Brian Mowll, "Toxic Connection to Diabetes and Metabolic Syndrome," Diabetes Summit 2018, April 23–30, 2018.

5   Colbert, *Toxic Relief*, 6.

6   Dr. Mark Stengler interview with Mark Hyman, "Cancer Detox: Understanding the Root Cause of Cancer," *Beyond Chemo,* May 16, 2018.

7   Environmental Protection Agency, "2012 Toxic Release Inventory National Analysis Overview," www.epa.gov/sites/production/files/2014-01/documents/1-exec_sum_2012_tri_na_overview_document_0.pdf (accessed January 16, 2019).

8   Joe Mercola, "Common Chemicals Threaten Male Fertility," *Mercola*, June 4, 2009, https://articles.mercola.com/sites/articles/archive/2009/06/04/common-chemicals-threaten-male-fertility.aspx (accessed January 16, 2019).

9   Colbert, *Toxic Relief*, 17.

10 Woodson Merrill, "Why You Should Detox with Whole Foods," *The Dr. Oz Show,* October 21, 2014, www.doctoroz.com/episode/plan-detox-without-juicing (accessed January 16, 2019).

11 "Body Burden: The Pollution in Newborns," *Environmental Working Group*, July 24, 2005, www.ewg.org/research/body-burden-pollution-newborns# (accessed January 16, 2019).

12   Ty Bollinger, "The Truth About Detox," *The Truth About Cancer*, https:// thetruthaboutdetox.com/1/insider-access/ (accessed January 17, 2019).

13   Laura Reiley, "The Organic Food Industry Is Booming, and That May Be Bad for Consumers," *The Washington Post*, March 14, 2019.

14   Alena Hall, "What Happened after One Family Went Organic for Just Two Weeks," *The Huffington Post*, May 15, 2015, www.huffingtonpost. com/2015/05/14/the-organic-effect_n_7244000.html (accessed January 17, 2019).

15   Joshua Axe, "Is Organic Really Better?" *Dr. Axe*, July 16, 2017, https://draxe. com/is-organic-really-better/ (accessed January 17, 2019).

16   "Organic Foods: Are They Safer? More Nutritious?" *Mayo Clinic*, April 4, 2018, www.mayoclinic.org/healthy-lifestyle/nutrition-and-healthy-eating/in-depth/ organic-food/art-20043880?pg=2 (accessed January 17, 2019).

17   "Exposure to Chemicals in Food," *BreastCancer.org*, www.breastcancer.org/risk/ factors/food_chem (accessed January 17, 2019).

18   Sonya Lunder, "EWG's 2019 Shopping Guide to Pesticides in Produce," *Environmental Working Group*, March 20, 2019, www.ewg.org/foodnews/ summary.php (accessed February 15, 2020).

19   Darryl Fears, "It's Not Just Flint. Lead Taints Water Across the U.S., EPA Records Show," *The Washington Post*, March 17, 2016.

20   Lindsay Oberst, "'Erin Brockovich' Carcinogen Found in the Drinking Water of More than 75% of Americans—Is Your Water Toxic?" *Food Revolution Network*, September 23, 2016, https://foodrevolution.org/blog/food-and-health/ chromium-6-in-drinking-water/ (accessed January 17, 2019).

21   Lindsay Oberst, "What You Need to Know about Bottled Water," *Food Revolution Network*, March 7, 2016, https://foodrevolution.org/blog/what-you-need-to-know-about-bottled-water/ (accessed January 17, 2019).

22   Leah Zerbe, "Top Bottled Water Risks: Are You Drinking This Toxic Rip-Off?" *Dr. Axe*, March 15, 2018, https://draxe.com/bottled-water-risks/ (accessed January 17, 2019).

23   Martin Wagner, Michael P. Schlüsener, Thomas A. Ternes, Jörg Oehlmann, "Identification of Putative Steroid Receptor Antagonists in Bottled Water: Combining Bioassays and High-Resolution Mass Spectrometry," *PLOS ONE*, August 28, 2013, https://doi.org/10.1371/journal.pone.0072472 (accessed January 17, 2019).

24   Martin Wagner and Jorg Oehlmann, "Endocrine Disruptors in Bottled Mineral Water: Estrogenic Activity in the E-Screen," *The Journal of Steroid Biochemistry and Molecular Biology* 127, no. 1-2 (October 2011): 128–135.

25   Martin Wagner and Jorg Oehlmann, "Endocrine Disruptors in Bottled Water: Total Estrogenic Burden and Migration from Plastic Bottles," *Environmental Science and Pollution Research* 16, no. 3 (May 2009): 278–286.

26 "Harmful Chemicals Found in Bottled Water," *Environmental Working Group*, October 15, 2008, www.ewg.org/news/news-releases/2008/10/15/harmful-chemicals-found-bottled-water (accessed January 17, 2019).

27 Joseph Pizzorno, *The Toxin Solution* (New York: HarperCollins, 2017), 40.

28 EPA Indoor AirPlus brochure, *U.S. Environmental Protection Agency*, August 2014, www.epa.gov/sites/production/files/2014-08/documents/consumer_brochure.pdf (accessed January 17, 2019).

29 Mike Adams, "Health Ranger Lab Analysis Eposes 700+ Chemicals in Tide Laundry Pods," *Natural News*, January 31, 2018, www.naturalnews.com/2018-01-31-health-ranger-lab-analysis-exposes-700-chemicals-in-tide-laundry-pods-many-are-extremely-toxic-to-human-health-and-aquatic-life.html (accessed January 17, 2019).

30 David Jockers, "The Dangers of Root Canals," *DrJockers.com*, https://drjockers.com/root-canals/ (accessed January 19, 2019).

31 "Factors with Unclear Effects on Breast Cancer," *American Cancer Society*, September 6, 2017, www.cancer.org/cancer/breast-cancer/risk-and-prevention/factors-with-unclear-effects-on-breast-cancer-risk.html (accessed January 17, 2019).

32 Edward Group, III, "How Healing Works," *The Truth About Cancer* in Anaheim, California, October 12, 2019.

Chapter 12: Detoxing to Reduce Your Toxic Load

1 Thomas Levy address to 35th Annual Cancer Convention, "Vitamin C Antidote to all Known Toxins," *YouTube*, May 5, 2012, www.youtube.com/watch?v=GpptUsJFCEY (accessed January 17, 2019).

2 Ron Hunninghake interview with Chris Wark, "MD on the Anticancer Power of IV Vitamin C," *Chris Beat Cancer*, September 24, 2018, www.chrisbeatcancer.com/ron-hunninghake-md-on-the-anticancer-power-of-vitamin-c (accessed January 17, 2019).

3 Jennifer Brown, "High-Dose Vitamin C Proves Safe and Well-Tolerated in Brain and Lung Cancer Trials," *Iowa Now*, March 30, 2017, https://now.uiowa.edu/2017/03/high-dose-vitamin-c-proves-safe-and-well-tolerated-brain-and-lung-cancer-trials (accessed April 3, 2019).

4 Jihye Yun et al, "Vitamin C Selectively Kills KRAS and BRAF Mutant Colorectal Cancer Cells by Targeting GAPDH," *Science* 350, no. 6266 (December 11, 2015), 1391–1396.

5 Josh Goldstein, "High Dose Vitamin C for Advanced Pancreatic Cancer," *Thomas Jefferson University*, January 17, 2012, http://blogs.jefferson.edu/

atjeff/2012/01/17/high-dose-vitamin-c-for-advanced-pancreatic-cancer (accessed April 3, 2019).

6   Hunninghake, "MD on the Anticancer Power of IV Vitamin C."

7   David Jockers, "5 Healing Benefits of Intermittent Fasting, *DrJockers.com*, https://drjockers.com/5-healing-benefits-intermittent-fasting (accessed January 17, 2019).

8   Adapted from Laura Smith, *The 30-Day Faith Detox* (Bloomington: Chosen Books, 2016), 242.

Chapter 13: The Invisible Toxin

1   Julia Layton, "How does the body make electricity—and how does it use it?" *How Stuff Works*, https://health.howstuffworks.com/human-body/systems/nervous-system/human-body-make-electricity.htm (accessed March 20, 2019).

2   Devra Davis, "The Truth about Mobile Phone and Wireless Radiation," *YouTube*, December 2, 2015, www.youtube.com/watch?v=BwyDCHf5iCY&t=34s (accessed January 17, 2019).

3   IARC Press Release, "IARC Classifies Radiofrequency Electromagnetic Fields as Possibly Carcinogenic to Humans," *International Agency for Research on Cancer*, May 31, 2011, www.iarc.fr/en/media-centre/pr/2011/pdfs/pr208_E.pdf (accessed January 17, 2019).

4   Ashok Agarwal, Fnu Deepinder, Rakesh K. Sharma, Geetha Ranga, and Jianbo Li, "Effect of Cell Phone Usage on Semen Analysis in Men Attending Infertility Clinic: An Observational Study," *Fertility and Sterility* 89, no. 1 (January 2008): 124–128.

5   Lisa Bailey, "Cell Phones in Your Bra, Bad Idea!" *YouTube*, August 25, 2014, www.youtube.com/watch?v=e51F1iCx0mM (accessed January 17, 2019).

6   Lisa Bailey, "Skeptical About Cell Phones and Your Health?" *YouTube*, April 9, 2014, www.youtube.com/watch?v=IS8_OIEKVnk (accessed January 17, 2019).

7   Andrew Goldsworthy, "The Biological Effects of Weak Electromagnetic Fields," Stop Smart Meters brochure, March 2012, http://stopsmartmeters.org.uk/wp-content/uploads/2012/04/Biol-Effects-EMFs-2012-NZ1.pdf (accessed January 17, 2019).

8   Devra Davis, "The Truth about Mobile Phone and Wireless Radiation."

9   Martin Blank, "BioInitiative Report: A Rational for Biologically-Based Exposure Standards for Low-Intensity Electromagnetic Radiation," *BioInitiative 2012*, https://bioinitiative.org (accessed January 17, 2019).

10   Jeromy Johnson, "Wireless Wake-Up Call," www.youtube.com/watch?v=F0NEaPTu9oI (accessed April 6, 2019).

Chapter 14: Restoring Your Microbiome

1   Raphael Kellman, "The Microbiome and Autoimmune Disease," interview with Dr. Peter Osbourne, *Autoimmune Revolution*, February 3, 2017.

2   Tom O'Bryan, "How to Heal the Gut," *Solving Leaky Gut*, https://solvingleakygut. com/dr-tom-gut-presentation (accessed January 17, 2019).

3   Michael Murray, Digestive Summit, September 12, 2017.

4   G. Vighi, F. Marcucci, L. Sensi, G. Di Cara, and F. Frati, "Allergy and the Gastrointestinal System," *National Center for Biotechnology Information*, www. ncbi.nlm.nih.gov/pmc/articles/PMC2515351 (accessed July 15, 2019).

5   Raphael Kellman, "10 Things You Need to Know About Your Microbiome," *mindbodygreen*, www.mindbodygreen.com/0-14119/10-things-you-need-to-know-about-your-microbiome.html (accessed January 17, 2019).

6   Russell Jaffe, "Predictive Biomarkers for Digestive Health in the 21st Century," interview with Michael Murray, Digestive Summit, September 12, 2017.

7   Brian Mowll, "The Little-Known Link Between Diabetes and the Gut," Digestive Health Summit, September 13, 2017.

8   Ritamarie Loscalzo, "How Insulin Resistance Is Tied to Digestion," Digestive Health Summit, September 14, 2017.

9   "Chronic Inflammation," *National Cancer Institute*, April 29, 2015, www. cancer.gov/about-cancer/causes-prevention/risk/chronic-inflammation (accessed January 17, 2019).

10   Safia Danovi, "Feeling the Heat—the Link Between Inflammation and Cancer, *Cancer Research UK*, February 1, 2013, http://scienceblog.cancerresearchuk. org/2013/02/01/feeling-the-heat-the-link-between-inflammation-and-cancer (accessed January 17, 2019).

11   Jillian Levy, "Gut Bacteria Benefits: Could Better Bacteria Actually Cure Your Condition?" *Dr. Axe*, October 23, 2016, https://draxe.com/gut-bacteria-benefits (accessed January 17, 2019).

12   Marcelo Campos, "Leaky Gut: What Is It, and What Does It Mean for You?" *Harvard Health Publishing*, www.health.harvard.edu/blog/leaky-gut-what-is-it-and-what-does-it-mean-for-you-2017092212451 (accessed March 22, 2019).

13   Thomas Jefferson University, "Stronger Intestinal Barrier May Prevent Cancer in the Rest of the Body, New Study Suggests," *Science Daily*, February 21, 2012, www.sciencedaily.com/releases/2012/02/120221212345.htm (accessed January 17, 2019).

14   O'Bryan, "How to Heal the Gut" presentation.

15   Ibid.

16   Peter Osborne, "Autoimmune Recovery: Pulling the Pieces Together," *Autoimmune Revolution*, January 16, 2017.

17   Josh Axe, "The Leaky Gut Diet and Treatment Plan," *Dr. Axe*, July 30, 2018, https://draxe.com/4-steps-to-heal-leaky-gut-and-autoimmune-disease (accessed January 17, 2019).

18   Ibid.

19   Kristina Campbell, "Dr. Allan Walker, on the Harvard Probiotics Symposium," *Gut Microbiota for Health*, October 13, 2014, www.gutmicrobiotaforhealth.com/en/dr-allan-walker-on-the-harvard-probiotics-symposium (accessed January 17, 2019).

20   Daniel Pompa, "It's Not Just Gluten—The Glyphosate Threat," *Pompa*, January 28, 2015, https://drpompa.com/fasting-diet/glyphosate-threat-its-not-just-gluten (accessed January 17, 2019).

21   Stephanie Seneff, "The Dangers of Glyphosate," *Pompa*, January 5, 2016, https://drpompa.com/cellular-health/the-dangers-of-glyphosate-an-interview-with-dr-stephanie-seneff (accessed January 17, 2019).

22   Ocean Robbins, "What the $289 Million Verdict Against Monsanto Means to You," *Food Revolution Network*, August 24, 2018, https://foodrevolution.org/blog/monsanto-lawsuit-dewayne-johnson/ (accessed January 17, 2019).

23   American Cancer Society, "Known and Probable Carcinogens," *American Cancer Society*, www.cancer.org/cancer/cancer-causes/general-info/known-and-probable-human-carcinogens.html (accessed January 17, 2019).

24   Andy Coglan, "More Than Half of the EU Officially Bans Genetically Modified Crops," *New Scientist*, October 2015, www.newscientist.com/article/dn28283-more-than-half-of-european-union-votes-to-ban-growing-gm-crops? (accessed January 17, 2019).

25   "France's Macron Vows to Bran Glyphosate Weed Killer, as Germany Swings EU Vote in Its Favor," *RT News*, November 28, 2017, www.rt.com/news/411135-france-ban-monsanto-germany-vote (accessed January 18, 2019).

26   Geoffrey Mohan, "California Lists Roundup Ingredient as a Chemical Linked to Cancer; Monsanto Vows to Fight, *Los Angeles Times*, June 27, 2017, www.latimes.com/business/la-fi-roundup-cancer-20170626-story.html   (accessed January 18, 2019).

27   Tina Bellon, "Monsanto Ordered to Pay $289 Million in World's First Roundup Cancer Trial," *Reuters*, August 10, 2018, www.reuters.com/article/us-monsanto-cancer-lawsuit/monsanto-ordered-to-pay-289-million-in-worlds-first-roundup-cancer-trial-idUSKBN1KV2HB_(accessed January 18, 2019).

28   Sam Levin, "Monsanto 'Bullied Scientists' and Hid Weedkiller Cancer Risk, Lawyer Tells Court," *The Guardian*, July 9, 2018, www.theguardian.com/business/2018/jul/09/monsanto-trial-roundup-weedkiller-cancer-dewayne-johnson (accessed January 18, 2019).

29   Ludwig Burger, "Bayer's Monsanto Faces 8,000 Lawsuits on Glyphosate," *Reuters*, August 23, 2018, www.reuters.com/article/us-bayer-glyphosate-lawsuits/

bayers-monsanto-faces-8000-lawsuits-on-glyphosate-idUSKCN1L81J0 (accessed January 18, 2019).

30 Mercedes Clemente-Postigo, Maria Isabel Queipo-Ortuño, Maria Boto-Ordoñez, Leticia Coin-Aragüez, Maria del Mar Roca-Rodriguez, Javier Delgado-Lista, Fernando Cardona, Cristina Andres-Lacueva, Francisco J Tinahones, "Effect of Acute and Chronic Red Wine Consumption on Lipopolysaccharide Concentration," *The American Journal of Clinical Nutrition* 97, no. 5 (May 1, 2019) 1053-61, https://doi.org/10.3945/ajcn.112.051128 (accessed January 18, 2019).

31 Maria Queido-Ortuno, Maria Boto-Ordoñez, Mora Murri, Juan Miguel Gomez-Zumaquero, Mercedes Clemente-Postigo, Ramon Estruch, Fernando Cardona Diaz, Cristina Andrés-Lacueva, Francisco J Tinahones, "Influence of Red Wine Polyphenols and Ethanol on the Gut Microbiota Ecology and Biochemical Biomarkers," *American Journal of Clinical Nutrition* 95, no. 6 (June 1, 2012): 1323–1334.

32 David Perlmutter, "Fill Your Glass with This to Improve Gut Microbiota," *David Perlmutter MD*, September 2, 2014, www.drperlmutter.com/cheers-red-wine/ (accessed January 18, 2019).

Chapter 15: For Breast and Estrogen-Fed Cancer Only

1 "Breast Cancer Facts," *National Breast Cancer Foundation*, www.nationalbreastcancer.org/breast-cancer-facts (accessed January 18, 2019).

2 Aleksandra Fucic, Marija Gamulin, Zeljko Ferencic, Jelena Katic, Martin Krayer von Krauss, Alena Bartonova, and Domenico F Merlo, "Environmental Exposure to Xenoestrogens and Oestrogen-Related Cancers: Reproductive System, Breast, Lung, Kidney, Pancreas, and Brain," *Environmental Health* 11, no. 1 (June 28, 2012).

3 Pendergrast, *Breast Cancer*, 108.

4 The Collaborative Group on Hormonal Factors in Breast Cancer, "Breast Cancer and Hormonal Contraceptives: Collaborative Reanalysis of Individual Data on 53,297 Women with Breast Cancer and 100,239 Women without Breast Cancer from 54 Epidemiological Studies," *The Lancet* 347, no. 9017 (June 22, 1996): 1713–1727.

5 Veronique Desauliers, "The Surprising Reasons Male Breast Cancer Is on the Rise," *The Truth About Cancer*, June 17, 2016, https://thetruthaboutcancer.com/male-breast-cancer (accessed January 18, 2019).

6 Michal Melamed, Enrique Castaño, Angelo C. Notides, and Shlomo Sasson, "Molecular and Kinetic Basis for the Mixed Agonist/Antagonist Activity of Estriol," *Molecular Endocrinology* 11, no. 12 (November 1, 1997): 1868–1978.

7   Henry Lemon, Pradeep F. Kumar, Cary Peterson, Jorge F. Rodriguez-Sierra, and Katherine M. Abbo, "Inhibition of Radiogenic Mammary Carcinoma in Rats by Estriol or Tamoxifen," *Cancer* 63, no. 9 (May 1, 1989): 1685–1692.

8   David Jockers, "Finding Your Estrogen Quotient and Its Relationship to Cancer Risk," *Natural News*, May 12, 2014, www.naturalnews.com/045080_estrogen_quotient_cancer_risk_endocrine_system.html (accessed January 19, 2019).

9   Desaulniers, *Heal Breast Cancer Naturally*, 122.

10 Pendergrast, *Breast Cancer*, 27.

11 Christiane Northrup, "What are the Symptoms of Estrogen Dominance?" *Christiane Northrup MD*, February 6, 2007, www.drnorthrup.com/estrogen-dominance (accessed January 19, 2019).

12 Pendergrast, *Breast Cancer*, 114.

13 Yan Jiang, Yong Pan, Patrea R. Rhea, Lin Tan, Mihai Gagea, Lorenzo Cohen, Susan M. Fischer, and Peiying Yang, "A Sucrose-Enriched Diet Promotes Tumorigenesis in Mammary Gland in Part Through the 12-Lipoxygenase Pathway," *Cancer Research* 76, no. 1 (January 2016): 24–29.

14 Sayer Ji, "70 Reasons to Eat More Flaxseed," *Green Med Info*, August 11, 2018, www.greenmedinfo.com/blog/70-reasons-eat-more-flaxseed-1 (accessed January 19, 2019).

15 Lillian Thompson, Jian Min Chen, Tong Li, Kathrin Strasser-Weippl, and Paul E. Goss, "Dietary Flaxseed Alters Tumor Biological Markers in Postmenopausal Breast Cancer," *American Association for Cancer Research* 11, no. 10 (May 15, 2005): 3828–3836.

16 David Jockers, "Estrogen Dominance Symptoms and Solutions," *DrJockers.com*, May 19, 2018, https://drjockers.com/estrogen-dominance-symptoms (accessed January 19, 2019).

17 Ibid.

18 Brownstein, *Iodine*, 171.

19 Ibid.

20 William J. Mayo, "Susceptibility to Cancer," *Annals of Surgery* 93, no. 1 (January 1931): 16–19.

21 Salete Rios, Ana Carolina Rios Chen, Juliana Rios Chen, and Carlos Marino Calvano Filho, "Wearing a Tight Bra for Many Hours a Day Is Associated with Increased Risk of Breast Cancer," (September 2016), https://doi.org/10.13140/RG.2.2.10742.19525 (accessed January 19, 2019).

22 Sydney Singer and Soma Grismaijer, *Dressed to Kill*, 2nd edition, (New York: Square One, 2017). For more information, check out https://brasandbreastcancer.org/supportive-references.

23 "Why It's Important to Know if You Have Dense Breasts," *Cancer Treatment Centers of America*, January 3, 2017, www.cancercenter.com/discussions/blog/

why-its-important-to-know-if-you-have-dense-breasts (accessed January 20, 2019).

24 "New American Cancer Society Breast Cancer Screening Guidelines Start at 45," *BreastCancer.org*, www.breastcancer.org/research-news/acs-guidelines-recommend-mammograms-at-45 (accessed January 20, 2019).

Chapter 16: Promoting Longevity while Anticipating Heaven

1 Lynch, *Dirty Genes*, 29.

2 Michael Devitt, "CDC Data Show U.S. Life Expectancy Continues to Decline," *American Academy of Family Physicians*, www.aafp.org/news/health-of-the-public/20181210lifeexpectdrop.html (accessed March 29, 2018).

3 Thomas Bodenheimer, Ellen Chen, and Heather D. Bennett, "Confronting the Growing Burden of Chronic Disease," *Health Affairs* 98, no. 1 (January/February 2009).

4 "Nearly 1 in 5 People Have a Disability in the U.S., Census Bureau Reports," *United States Census Bureau*, July 25, 2012, www.census.gov/newsroom/releases/archives/miscellaneous/cb12-134.html (accessed January 20, 2019).

5 Leigh Erin Connealy, "The Cancer Revolution," *The Truth About Cancer* in Anaheim, California, October 13, 2019.

6 "Science Surgery: 'Do we all have potentially cancerous cells in our bodies?'" *Cancer Research UK*, https://scienceblog.cancerresearchuk.org/2018/04/18/science-surgery-do-we-all-have-potentially-cancerous-cells-in-our-bodies (accessed March 29, 2019).

Afterword: She Had to Find It Out for Herself

1 Ginny Dent Brant, "An Honest and Inspiring Interview with Joni Eareckson Tada," *Sonoma Christian Home*, May 5, 2013, https://sonomachristianhome.com/2013/05/an-honest-and-inspiring-interview-with-joni-eareckson-tada (accessed January 16, 2019).

2 James Forsythe, "The Cancer Solution that works 34X Better than Chemo," *The Christian Medical Science Summit*, September 18, 2019.

Milton Keynes UK
Ingram Content Group UK Ltd.
UKHW030854131024
449552UK00004B/102